HbA₁c in Diabetes
case studies using IFCC units

Edited by

Stephen Gough
Professor of Medicine
Institute of Biomedical Research
University of Birmingham
and Consultant Physician/Diabetologist, University Hospital
Birmingham NHS Foundation Trust
Birmingham, UK

Susan Manley
Clinical Biochemistry
University Hospital Birmingham NHS Foundation Trust
Birmingham, UK

Irene Stratton
English National Screening Programme for Diabetic
Retinopathy
Gloucestershire Hospitals NHS Foundation Trust
Cheltenham, UK

Diabetes
UK

The charity for
people with diabetes

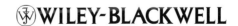

WILEY-BLACKWELL

This edition first published 2010, © 2010 by Blackwell Publishing Ltd

Blackwell Publishing was acquired by John Wiley & Sons in February 2007. Blackwell's publishing program has been merged with Wiley's global Scientific, Technical and Medical business to form Wiley-Blackwell.

Registered office: John Wiley & Sons Ltd, The Atrium, Southern Gate, Chichester, West Sussex, PO19 8SQ, UK

Editorial offices: 9600 Garsington Road, Oxford, OX4 2DQ, UK
      The Atrium, Southern Gate, Chichester, West Sussex, PO19 8SQ, UK
      111 River Street, Hoboken, NJ 07030-5774, USA

For details of our global editorial offices, for customer services and for information about how to apply for permission to reuse the copyright material in this book please see our website at www.wiley.com/wiley-blackwell

Library of Congress Cataloging-in-Publication Data

HbA1c in diabetes : case studies using IFCC units / edited by Stephen Gough, Susan Manley & Irene Stratton.
  p. ; cm.
  ISBN 978-1-4443-3444-9
  1. Diabetes--Great Britain. 2. Glycosylated hemoglobin--Measurement. I. Gough, Stephen, Ph. D.
II. Manley, Susan. III. Stratton, Irene. [DNLM: 1. International Federation of Clinical Chemistry and Laboratory Medicine. 2. Diabetes Mellitus--blood--Great Britain. 3. Blood Chemical Analysis--Great Britain. 4. Diabetes Mellitus--blood--Great Britain--Case Reports. 5. Hemoglobin A, Glycosylated--analysis--Great Britain. WK 810 H431 2010]
  RA645.D5H353 2010
  616.4'62--dc22

2009046374

ISBN: 9781444334449

A catalogue record for this book is available from the British Library.

Set in 9.5/12pt Minion by Sparks – www.sparkspublishing.com
Printed and bound in Singapore by Ho Printing Singapore Pte Ltd

1 2010

Contents

Contributor list

G. Pooler R. Archbold, Consultant Chemical Pathologist, Belfast, Northern Ireland, UK

Jane Armitage, Professor of Clinical Trials and Epidemiology, Oxford, UK

Timothy G. Barrett, Professor of Paediatric Endocrinology, Birmingham, UK

Varadarajan Baskar, Consultant Physician, Wolverhampton, UK

Rikke Borg, Research Fellow, Steno Diabetes Centre, Gentofte, Denmark

Jackie Carr-Smith, Research Nurse, Birmingham, UK

Lis Chandler, Research Nurse, Birmingham, UK

Chris Cottrell, Diabetes Specialist Nurse, Llanelli, Wales, UK

Robert Cramb, Consultant Chemical Pathologist, Birmingham, UK

Steven Creely, Specialist Registrar in Diabetes and Endocrinology, Birmingham, UK

Sean F. Dinneen, Consultant Physician, Galway, Ireland

Pamela Dyson, Dietician, Oxford, UK

Julie A. Edge, Consultant in Paediatric Diabetes, Oxford, UK

Adele Farnsworth, Lead Diabetic Retinal Screener, Birmingham, UK

Valeria Frighi, Senior Clinical Researcher, University of Oxford, UK

Andrea Gomes, MSc Student, Birmingham, UK

Helen Green, Diabetes Specialist Nurse, Llanelli, Wales, UK

Sarah Griffiths, Senior House Officer in Diabetes, Birmingham, UK

Daniel Hammersley, Medical Student, London, UK

Maggie Sinclair Hammersley, Consultant Physician, Oxford, UK

Richard Haynes, Clinical Research Fellow, Oxford, UK

Simon Heller, Professor of Clinical Diabetes, Sheffield, UK

R. Welby Henry, Consultant Physician, Belfast, Northern Ireland, UK

Laura Hikin, MSc Student, Birmingham, UK

Richard I. G. Holt, Professor in Diabetes and Endocrinology, Southampton, UK

W. Garry John, Consultant Clinical Biochemist, Norfolk and Norwich University Hospitals, Norwich, UK

M. Ali Karamat, Clinical Lecturer in Diabetes and Endocrinology, Birmingham, UK

Hamza Ali Khan, Specialist Registrar, Belfast, Northern Ireland, UK

Eric S. Kilpatrick, Honorary Professor in Clinical Biochemistry, Hull, UK

R. David Leslie, Professor of Diabetes and Autoimmunity, Queen Mary University of London, UK

Nick Lewis-Barned, Consultant Physician and Senior Lecturer, Northumbria, UK

Ernesto Lopez, Medical Student, London, UK

David R. McCance, Honorary Professor of Endocrinology/Consultant Physician, Royal Victoria Hospital, Belfast, Northern Ireland, UK

John A. McKnight, Consultant Physician, Western General Hospital, and Honorary Reader, University of Edinburgh, Scotland, UK

Ciara McLaughlin, Specialist Registrar, Royal Victoria Hospital, Belfast, Northern Ireland, UK

Susan E. Manley, Clinical Scientist, Birmingham, UK

Sally M. Marshall, Professor of Diabetes, Newcastle upon Tyne, UK

Sarah Moore, GP, Worcestershire, UK

Joanne Morling, Specialty Registrar in Public Health, University of Edinburgh, Scotland, UK

Parth Narendran, Clinical Senior Lecturer and Honorary Consultant in Diabetes, Birmingham, UK

Ailish G. Nugent, Consultant Physician, Belfast, Northern Ireland, UK

Máire O'Donnell, Research Associate, Galway, Ireland

Katharine R. Owen, Clinician Scientist, Oxford, UK

Richard Paisey, Consultant Physician, Torbay, UK

Stuart A. Ritchie, Specialist registrar, Edinburgh, Scotland, UK

Jonathan Roland, Consultant Diabetologist, Peterborough, UK

Rachel Round, Researcher, Birmingham, UK

Peter H. Scanlon, Consultant Ophthalmologist, Cheltenham and Oxford, UK

Ken Sikaris, Director of Chemical Pathology, Melbourne Pathology, Victoria, Australia

Janet Smith, Honorary Consultant Clinical Scientist, University Hospital Birmingham, UK/Honorary Senior Clinical Lecturer, Medical School, University of Birmingham, UK

Matthew Stephenson, Consultant Psychiatrist in Learning Disability, Oxford Learning Disability NHS Trust, Oxford, UK

Roy Taylor, Professor of Medicine and Metabolism, Newcastle upon Tyne, UK

Athinyaa Thiraviaraj, Specialist Registrar, Belfast, Northern Ireland, UK

Tara Wallace, Consultant Physician, Norfolk and Norwich University Hospitals, Norwich, UK

Jonathan Webber, Consultant Physician, Birmingham, UK

Amanda Webster, Genetic Diabetes Specialist Nurse, Oxford, UK

Rob Willox, Retinal Screening Technician, Torbay, UK

Alex Wright, Consultant Physician, Walsall/Birmingham, and Honorary Senior Lecturer, Birmingham, UK

You Yi Hong, Surgical Intern, Galway, Ireland

Preface

The measurement of HbA_{1c} is a key tool in the treatment of diabetes mellitus. For health care professionals involved in the management of diabetes in the UK there is an additional complication, between 2009 and 2011, with a change of HbA_{1c} units. The old DCCT percentage is giving way to the internationally recognised IFCC units of mmol/mol in 2011.

To further the understanding of HbA_{1c} measurements, we have summarised the important issues and then appended a number of case studies involving a wide range of patients from children to the elderly, showing the measurements in both the 'old' and 'new' units. These cover a wide range of diabetes-related conditions and describe the treatment plans and follow-up. We hope that this book will be a useful resource for all those involved in diabetes care as they come to terms with IFCC reporting.

This cannot be the last word on the measurement or role of HbA_{1c} and we look forward to continuing the interaction with colleagues in the UK and further afield.

Stephen Gough, Susan Manley, Irene Stratton
Birmingham, UK

Acknowledgements

We are most grateful to all the contributors who have given us the benefit of their experience and to their patients, and also to Professor Sir George Alberti and Diabetes UK for their endorsement of the book. We also wish to thank Vivienne Kendall for assembling the case studies, Alison Barratt for designing the cover and the staff at Wiley-Blackwell for their help with the editorial and production processes. In addition, we thank Keith Chambers, Jonathan Middle, Peter Nightingale, Marco Ossani, Francesco Pessala, Janet Smith and the biomedical scientists at University Hospital Birmingham NHS Foundation Trust. We acknowledge receipt of a grant from the Novo Nordisk Educational Research Foundation for our research study, the NOVO GFH (glucose, fructosamine and HbA_{1c}) Study.

The following have kindly given their permission for us to use previously published material:

Rikke Borg (Figure 2); Keith Chambers (Figure 5); Rury Holman (Figure 6; unpublished and reproduced with permission); *The Lancet* (1998) 352, 837–53 and *NEJM* (2008) 359, 1577–89 (Figures 7A and B); *BMJ* (2000) 321, 405–12 (Figure 8); *NEJM* (1993) 329, 977–86 (Figure 9); *Diabetic Medicine* (2009) 26,115–21 (Figure 10); Ken Sikaris (Figure 11); *Diabetes Care* (2008) 31, 1473–78 (Figure 12); poster from the GFH Study at IDF 2009 (Figure 14); Garry John (Figure 15; unpublished and reproduced with permission); *UK Office of Public Sector Information: Health Technology Assessment* (2000) 4 (3); Reproduced under the terms of Click Use PSI Licence C2009002437 (Figure 16); Clinical Biochemistry, University Hospital Birmingham NHS Foundation Trust (Figure 17); *Ann Clin Biochem* (2006) 43, 135–45. Copyright (2006) Royal Society of Medicine Press, UK (Figure 18); Jonathan Middle, NEQAS (Figure 19); Becton Dickinson (Figure 20); Medtronic (Figure 21); plates reproduced with permission from patients, the South Devon Healthcare Trust and the Gloucestershire Hospitals NHS Foundation Trust. Our thanks also to Judith Kuenen for help in developing Table 1.

Foreword

The relation of glycated haemoglobin to blood glucose levels was first discovered about 40 years ago. Over the next decade assays were developed to allow its routine use. It was a massive breakthrough for people with diabetes and health professionals, as for the first time there was an independent way of assessing average blood glucose levels over a period of several weeks. The test was first used for assessing control in 1976, and a wide range of different tests were developed. Some of these were cumbersome; many gave different values and it was not until the DCCT trial that an effort was made to standardise reporting. Since then, many laboratories worldwide align their results against the DCCT standard. The results have traditionally been presented as a percentage of total haemoglobin.

In the interim, the IFCC has developed a new standard and reference method against which other methods can be standardised, and absolute amounts of HbA_{1c} can be measured. As a result the recommendation now is that results should be presented as mmol glycated haemoglobin/mol unglycated haemoglobin. The UK is following this recommendation; parallel reporting is now in place and will continue until mid-2011. Obviously the numbers are different and it will take time for professionals and patients to attune themselves to the new units. This is of course not a new problem. Thirty-five years ago, most clinical biochemistry results were changed from a weight-based system to a molar system, and many analytes – including glucose – showed large changes in the actual numbers reported. The switch, backed by a strong educational program and initial double reporting, was relatively trouble-free.

The same should be true for HbA_{1c}. The current volume is an excellent adjunct to the educational process – and a novel and readable way of helping people. A series of case studies is presented, in which both ways of expressing HbA_{1c} are used. This covers a wide range of values and through repetition, the numbers start to become more familiar and make sense.

KGMM Alberti
St Mary's Hospital, London

List of abbreviations

AA	Normal haemoglobin
AC	Haemoglobin C trait
ACB	Association for Clinical Biochemistry
ACD	Antihypertensive ACD algorithm
ACE	Angiotensin-converting enzyme
ACR	Albumin creatinine ratio
ACTH	Adrenocorticotropic hormone
AD	Haemoglobin D trait
ADA	American Diabetes Association
ADAG	A1C-derived average glucose
AE	Haemoglobin E trait
ALP	Alkaline phosphatase
ALT	Alanine aminotransferase
ARB	Adrenergic receptor blocker
AS	Sickle cell trait
A1C	HbA_{1c}
BHS	British Hypertension Society
BM	Blood glucose strips
BMI	Body mass index
CGM	Continuous blood glucose monitoring
CSII	Continuous subcutaneous insulin infusion
DCCT	Diabetes Control and Complications Trial
DIGAMI	Diabetes Mellitus, Insulin–Glucose Infusion in Acute Myocardial Infarction
DM	Diabetes mellitus
DUK	Diabetes UK
DVT	Deep vein thrombosis
eAG	Estimated average glucose
EASD	European Association for the Study of Diabetes
ECG	Electrocardiogram
EDTA	Ethylenediamine tetraacetic acid
eGFR	Estimated glomerular filtration rate
FBG	Fasting blood glucose
FPG	Fasting plasma glucose
FSH	Follicle stimulating hormone
GAD	Glutamic acid decarboxylase
GFH	Glucose Fructosamine HbA_{1c} (research study)

Hb	Haemoglobin
HbA$_{1c}$	Glycated haemoglobin
HbF	Fetal haemoglobin
HDL	High-density lipoprotein
HNF1A	Hepatic nuclear factor 1A
HPLC	High performance liquid chromatography
IDF	International Diabetes Foundation
IFCC	International Federation of Clinical Chemistry and Laboratory Medicine
IFG	Impaired fasting glucose
IGF-1	Insulin-like growth factor 1
IGT	Impaired glucose tolerance
JDS	Japanese Diabetes Society
LDL	Low-density lipoprotein
LH	Luteinising hormone
MODY	Maturity onset diabetes of the young
MRI	Magnetic resonance imaging
NGSP	National Glycohemoglobin Standardization Program
NICE	National Institute for Health and Clinical Excellence
OGTT	Oral glucose tolerance test
PCI	Percutaneous coronary intervention (angioplasty)
POCT	Point of care testing
RPG	Random plasma glucose
SI	Système Internationale
SMBG	Self monitoring of blood glucose
SS	Sickle cell disease/anaemia
T$_4$	Thyroxine
TSH	Thyroid-stimulating hormone
UKPDS	UK Prospective Diabetes Study
VA	Visual acuity
WHO	World Health Organisation
2hPG	2 hour plasma glucose
^{32}P	Radioactive isotope of phosphorus

Introduction

Background

What is diabetes?

Impairment of glucose regulation in the body leads to diabetes. In untreated diabetes, glucose levels in the blood increase. In type 1 diabetes, mainly found in children and young adults, β-cells in the islets of Langerhans of the pancreas fail to secrete insulin and insulin replacement is required.

In people with type 2 diabetes, typically diagnosed in middle age but now also in children, blood glucose levels rise as a result of both resistance to the action of insulin and also progressive β-cell dysfunction (Figure 1). In type 2 diabetes, treatment involves lifestyle changes and oral antidiabetes drugs that lead to an increase in insulin secretion from the pancreas or increased insulin sensitivity in the tissues. Injectable treatments may also be required, with the majority of people with type 2 diabetes ultimately requiring insulin.

Despite defects in the secretion and action of insulin being the cause of diabetes, the hormone is rarely measured in routine clinical care, although it can be measured easily on automated equipment in pathology laboratories. A reference method using mass spectrometry has been developed for calibration, so that in-

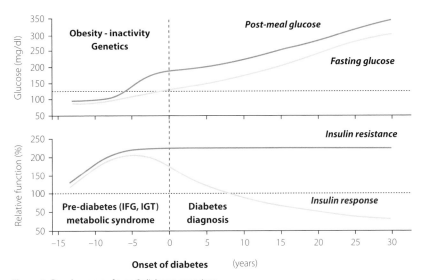

Figure 1 Development of type 2 diabetes over time.

sulin values obtained from different methods will be comparable. Blood glucose control is usually monitored in patients by determination of HbA$_{1c}$ – a measure of glucose-bound (glycated) haemoglobin. This is proportional to the amount of glucose in the blood over the previous two to three months, the lifespan of red blood cells. Lowering blood glucose levels will lead to lower HbA$_{1c}$ and failure to control blood glucose successfully, to high HbA$_{1c}$. Glycated haemoglobin has been used for assessing glycaemic control since 1976.

The prevalence of diabetes, particularly type 2, is increasing inexorably – putting a significant strain on healthcare resources that will impact most on developing regions of the world. Many of the ethnic groups that will be affected (e.g. those in India, China and Africa) are more susceptible to diabetes than Caucasians. Lifestyle is also a major factor: the likelihood of developing diabetes is increased when exercise levels are reduced and high calorific diets adopted, leading to overweight or obesity. These changes are typically related to urbanisation, industrialisation and the adoption of a western lifestyle.

The concentration of glucose in blood varies according to the time of the day and reflects the patient's nutritional intake and ability to metabolise glucose (Figure 2). In practice, blood is collected by health care professionals, with glucose measured at any time of the day (random plasma glucose, RPG), or at a pre-arranged time after fasting (fasting plasma glucose, FPG). Plasma glucose values are sometimes recorded at specified times, e.g. two hours after a meal or the time of the last meal is recorded.

Smaller differences occur in glucose levels when blood is obtained from various sites of the body or when different devices are used for measurement. Blood can be taken from veins (venous), finger pricks (capillary), the abdomen (interstitial) or arteries (arterial). To monitor their glucose control, patients may test their own blood using meters or implanted sensors. For medical review, they can have blood samples taken in a clinical setting, with measurement at point of care or in a central laboratory.

What is HbA$_{1c}$?

Glycation of haemoglobin is not catalysed by enzymes, but occurs through a chemical reaction that depends on the exposure of red blood cells to glucose circulating in the blood (Figure 3). Clinical management of diabetes involves regular measurement of HbA$_{1c}$ to monitor the glucose level in the bloodstream. HbA$_{1c}$ is usually measured at three- or six-monthly intervals or at the time of an annual review. One of the advantages of measuring HbA$_{1c}$ rather than glucose is that fasting is not required. Although a venous blood sample is required routinely by most laboratories, HbA$_{1c}$ can also be measured on capillary blood obtained from a finger prick, using smaller analysers located at point of care.

Any event or condition that affects haemoglobin, or red blood cells or their turnover may affect the amount of HbA$_{1c}$ in circulating blood. Measurement of reticulocytes (immature red blood cells) will determine whether the turnover of red blood cells is affected; if it is accelerated, the reticulocyte count will be

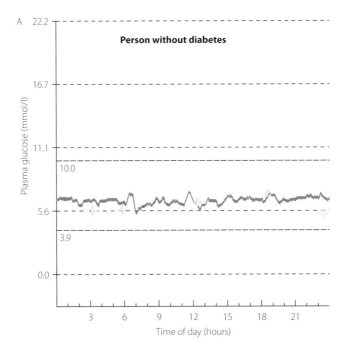

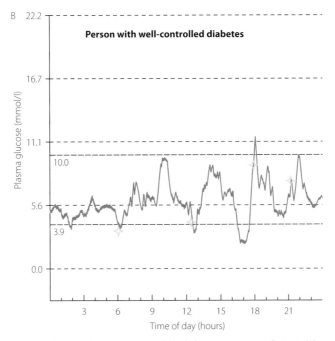

Figure 2 Daily profile from implanted continuous blood glucose monitoring device in (A) person without diabetes; (B) person with well-controlled type 1 diabetes.

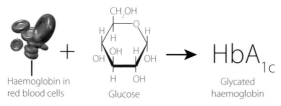

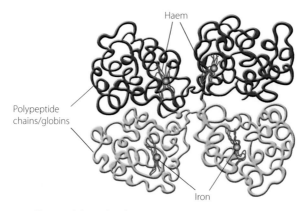

Figure 3 Formation of HbA₁c.

high. Some anaemias, e.g. haemolytic anaemia and polycythaemia rubra vera can depress HbA₁c, because the lifespan of the red blood cells is shorter than normal. Abnormal or variant haemoglobins may also affect HbA₁c results, as discussed later.

The haemoglobin molecule is composed of four globin protein chains, each with a haem moiety, held together by non-covalent interactions (Figure 4). The 3D structure of the molecule changes when oxygen binds to the haem. In normal adult haemoglobin (HbA), there are 2 α globin chains of 141 amino acids each, coded by DNA on chromosome 16, and 2 β globin chains of 146 amino acids coded on chromosome 11. Fetal haemoglobin, present in babies, binds oxygen with a greater affinity than adult haemoglobin; it contains 2 α chains and 2 γ chains coded on chromosome 11. The γ chain has less positive charges than the adult β chain. Over the first year of life, the production of fetal haemoglobin ceases so that it accounts for less than one per cent of haemoglobin in adults (Figure 5). In certain circumstances due to genetic abnormalities, higher amounts of fetal haemoglobin occur in adults (termed hereditary persistence of fetal haemoglobin) which can lead to problems when using HbA₁c to monitor glucose control in diabetes.

Figure 4 Structure of haemoglobin molecule.

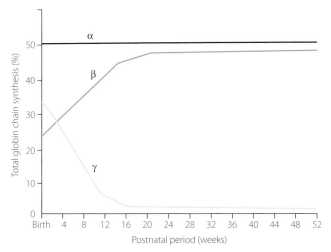

Figure 5 Development of adult haemoglobin.

The main component of glycated haemoglobin, HbA_{1c} is formed by the binding of glucose to the amino acid at the N-terminal of the β globin chain, valine. Initially a labile version of HbA_{1c} is formed, followed by a more stable version produced by a chemical process known as the Amadori rearrangement. Other glycated versions of haemoglobin with different glucose derivatives occur naturally, i.e. HbA_{1a} and HbA_{1b}. These glycated haemoglobins have different charges from HbA_{1c} which is useful when separating glycated haemoglobins for measurement of HbA_{1c}.

Abnormal (variant) haemoglobins, such as HbS (sickle cell), HbC, and HbD and the many others so far identified, have different amino acids sequences in the globin chains compared to normal haemoglobin HbA, caused by DNA mutations. High performance liquid chromatography (HPLC), used in biochemistry and haematology laboratories, can separate these haemoglobins according to their charge.

Recent research studies

Why is HbA_{1c} important?

The crucial importance of measuring HbA_{1c} has been shown by two important, large-scale, diabetes studies. Both of the major randomised controlled trials, the US Diabetes Control and Complications Trial (DCCT) and the UK Prospective Diabetes Study (UKPDS), showed that the use of intensive therapies for the reduction of blood glucose resulted in significant reductions in the risk of microvascular

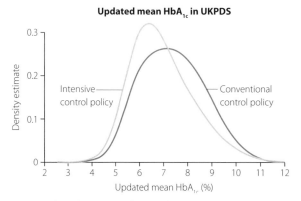

Figure 6 HbA$_{1c}$ in intensively and conventionally treated patients in the UKPDS.

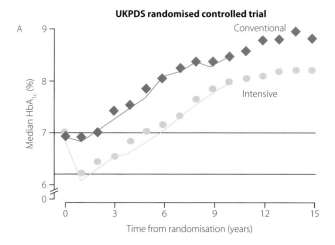

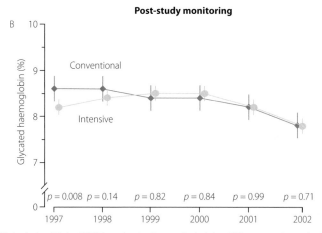

Figure 7 HbA$_{1c}$ during (A) the UKPDS randomised controlled trial and (B) post-study monitoring.

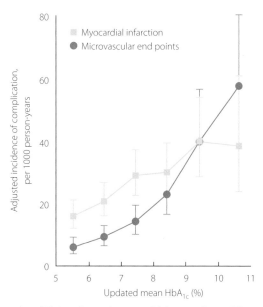

Figure 8 The relationship of HbA$_{1c}$ with complications of diabetes in the UKPDS.

complications of diabetes, as against the conventional therapy at that time. Intensive therapy resulted in a 2% lowering of HbA$_{1c}$ in the DCCT in patients with type 1 diabetes and 1% in the UKPDS for patients with type 2 diabetes (Figure 6).

In the UKPDS, HbA$_{1c}$ rose over time in both treatment groups, but not in the post-trial monitoring study when the treatment protocols were discontinued and all patients were treated to intensive targets (Figure 7). It should be noted that 'intensive treatment' in the trial conducted between 1977 and 1997 was not the same as that used in 2009.

The overall exposure of haemoglobin to glucose in the UKPDS presented as 'updated mean HbA$_{1c}$' was shown to be related to the incidence of complications found in the study (Figure 8). The mean updated HbA$_{1c}$ at any time point was the average up to that point in the study.

The UKPDS showed the relationships of updated mean HbA$_{1c}$ to retinopathy and macrovascular disease to be different. Low levels of HbA$_{1c}$ were related to a lower incidence of retinopathy than of macrovascular disease, with retinopathy increasing more steeply as HbA$_{1c}$ increased. Clearly it is important, when treating patients, to balance the lowering of HbA$_{1c}$ with an acceptable rate of hypoglycaemia for the particular patient (Figure 9).

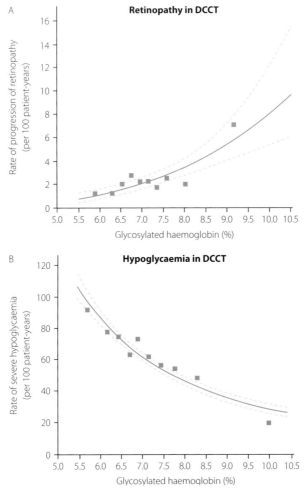

Figure 9 The relationship of HbA₁c with (A) retinopathy and (B) hypoglycaemia in the DCCT.

How does HbA₁c relate to glucose?

A graphical representation of the relationship of HbA₁c to FPG and 2 hour plasma glucose (2hPG) at the time of an oral glucose tolerance test (OGTT) was published in 2009 (Figure 10). This study included 1175 Australian patients referred for various reasons including impaired fasting glucose (IFG) identified by WHO criteria (i.e. FPG 6.1–6.9 mmol/l) which was detected in 26% of the population at OGTT. Venous blood samples were collected and spun within 30 minutes. Impaired glucose tolerance (IGT) was defined as 2hPG ≥7.8 and ≤11.1 mmol/l; and diabetes mellitus either FPG ≥7.0 mmol/l or 2hPG>11.1 mmol/l. Although the 2005 International Diabetes Federation (IDF) Clinical Guideline recommended that HbA₁c be measured when a patient attends for OGTT, it is only measured at OGTT in a minority of laboratories in the UK. People can be classified as having diabetes

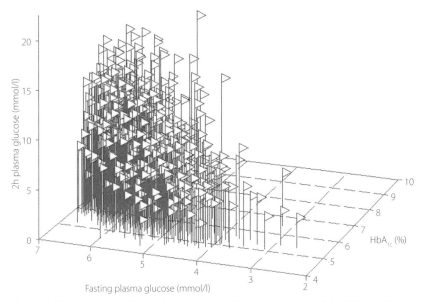

Figure 10 The relationship of fasting plasma glucose and 2h plasma glucose with HbA₁c in oral glucose tolerance test.

or pre-diabetes from plasma glucose measurements either (i) after fasting which identifies IFG or diabetes mellitus (DM) or (ii) from an OGTT which identifies IFG, impaired glucose tolerance (IGT) or DM. These two diagnostic methods do not necessarily lead to the same classification in an individual patient. In the UK, only patients with IFG are routinely referred for OGTT.

In the Australian cohort, the median HbA₁c for each group increased as the glycaemic category worsened, but there was considerable overlap in the HbA₁c for the different categories (Figure 11 overleaf). A similar pattern was observed in another cohort consisting of a more constrained population of 500 patients from the UK referred with IFG. About 10% of the UK population studied were South Asian; the others were mainly white Caucasian but some were Afro-Caribbean. Capillary blood samples were collected for measurement of HbA₁c and plasma glucose from the UK patients.

The recent international A1C-Derived Average Glucose (ADAG) Study, sponsored by the American Diabetes Association (ADA), the European Association for the Study of Diabetes (EASD) and IDF, involved over 600 participants in eleven countries. These included patients with type 1 or type 2 diabetes with stable control, and volunteers without diabetes. The relationship between 24-hour blood glucose (measured using implanted 24-hour monitoring devices and seven-point daily profiles from glucose meters) and HbA₁c was determined (Figure 12).

This study showed a closer relationship between glucose and HbA₁c data than other studies, due to 24-hour glucose monitoring and more frequent HbA₁c measurement. A Pearson correlation coefficient of $r = 0.92$ was obtained for the whole population. However, opinion is divided as to whether the scatter about the regres-

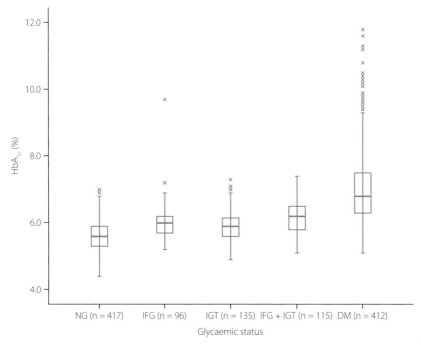

Figure 11 HbA$_{1c}$ by the category of glycaemia determined at OGTT (central line median, box IQ range).

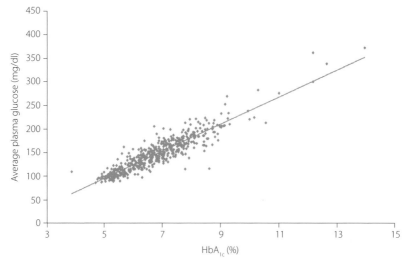

Figure 12 HbA$_{1c}$ and average plasma glucose measured over 24 hours in the ADAG study (180 mg/dl ≡ 10 mmol/l).

sion line is due to measurement error alone, or whether individual differences in the rate of glycation of haemoglobin are also involved. These data have been used to produce an estimated average glucose value (eAG) from the measured HbA$_{1c}$ – rather like estimated glomerular filtration rate (eGFR) which is obtained from

Table 1 Uncertainty about eAG derived from measured HbA$_{1c}$

HbA$_{1c}$		95% prediction interval (mmol/l)		
IFCC (mmol/mol)	DCCT (%)	eAG	Lower	Upper
42	6	7.0	5.5	8.5
53	7	8.5	6.8	10.3
64	8	10.1	8.1	12.1
75	9	11.6	9.4	13.9
86	10	13.2	10.7	15.7
97	11	14.8	12.0	17.5
108	12	16.3	13.3	19.3

measured serum creatinine. Because of these limitations, reporting of eAG, along with the actual HbA$_{1c}$ result, varies between countries (Table 1).

The researchers reported that the relationship between glucose and HbA$_{1c}$ was influenced only by the glucose concentration and length of exposure of red blood cells to glucose. The gender, age, type of diabetes or ethnicity of those studied (which did not include people from the Indian sub-continent due to technical problems) did not have any effect. However, reticulocytes and fructosamine were not measured for the study, nor was alcohol consumption recorded.

Research published in 2008 (Cohen *et al.*) has demonstrated that the survival of red blood cells varies sufficiently in haematologically normal people to cause clinically significant differences in HbA$_{1c}$. This could help to explain the discrepancy between HbA$_{1c}$ values in different patients with the same blood glucose levels.

HbA$_{1c}$ in clinical practice

How should HbA$_{1c}$ be reported?

HbA$_{1c}$ is measured in laboratories and at point of care using various chromatographic and immunological techniques, but only HPLC will detect the presence of abnormal haemoglobins. HbA$_{1c}$ has been reported in percentages aligned to the DCCT. A high-level reference method involving capillary electrophoresis and mass spectrometry is now available from the International Federation for Clinical Chemistry and Laboratory Medicine (IFCC) but is used only for calibration of HbA$_{1c}$ analysers, not for the measurement of patients' samples. DCCT-aligned HbA$_{1c}$ is converted into IFCC units using the following equation:

$$\text{IFCC-HbA}_{1c}\,(\text{mmol/mol}) \equiv [\text{DCCT-HbA}_{1c}\,(\%) - 2.15] \times 10.929.$$

In 2007, an international consensus committee of diabetes and clinical chemistry professionals recommended that HbA$_{1c}$ should be reported as follows:

- DCCT-aligned HbA$_{1c}$ as a percentage of unglycated haemoglobin (%)
- IFCC HbA$_{1c}$ as mmol glycated haemoglobin/mol unglycated haemoglobin (mmol/mol)

- eAG (estimated average glucose) derived from the relationship for HbA$_{1c}$ and glucose defined by the ADAG study (mmol/l or mg/dl, depending on the country concerned).

In the UK, it was decided to report IFCC units for HbA$_{1c}$ but not to report eAG because of the uncertainty around values derived for individual patients. Subsequently, the Department of Health, Diabetes UK (DUK) and the Association for Clinical Biochemistry (ACB) issued leaflets announcing that from 1 June 2009 until 31 May 2011, both DCCT-aligned HbA$_{1c}$ in % units and IFCC HbA$_{1c}$ in mmol/mol should be reported, and that from 1 June 2011, only IFCC HbA$_{1c}$ should be used (see ACB and DUK websites for leaflets).

When is HbA$_{1c}$ not appropriate?

In some circumstances HbA$_{1c}$ does not reflect blood glucose control. It is important that these are recognised; otherwise they could result in a patient being under- or over-treated. Usually these situations arise from coexisting medical conditions, such as haematological disorders, that affect red blood cells and haemoglobin turnover or its structure, renal or liver disease, and drugs or interventions that cause severe anaemia. Their effects on HbA$_{1c}$ are not well characterised but should be considered if a patient's HbA$_{1c}$ does not match their glucose measurements. Requesting a reticulocyte count, full blood count or identification of abnormal haemoglobin from a haematology department is desirable. A high reticulocyte count indicates the presence of immature red cells with a corresponding lowering of HbA$_{1c}$. Table 2 identifies circumstances in which HbA$_{1c}$ measurement is inappropriate.

Fructosamine is an alternative marker of glycaemic control that may be measured when HbA$_{1c}$ is inappropriate, or if measures of glycaemic control are required over a shorter time period. Fructosamine reflects the binding of glucose to plasma

Table 2 Circumstances affecting HbA$_{1c}$ values

After a blood transfusion
After venesection
Blood loss
Anaemias – polycythaemia rubra vera, sickle cell disease, haemolytic anaemia, post transplant anaemia, iron deficiency anaemia*
Presence of abnormal haemoglobins including fetal haemoglobin
Renal disease
Liver disease
Drugs that cause severe anaemia or affect red cell turnover, e.g. erythropoietin, some antiviral drugs
Excess alcohol intake associated with macrocytosis

* Causes an increase in HbA$_{1c}$

proteins (mainly albumin) and indicates the control of blood glucose over two to three weeks, the half-life of plasma albumin. It is measured on high-volume automated analysers in some, but not all, hospital laboratories and involves the reduction of a dye to produce a colour change.

If there is a suspicion that an HbA$_{1c}$ measurement does not accurately reflect a patient's glycaemic control, fructosamine measurement offers an alternative. However, fructosamine results will be lower if albumin turnover in the blood is increased, or if a patient has severe proteinuria and excretes large amounts of albumin, both glycated and unglycated, in their urine due to glomerular renal damage associated with diabetes. If the patient is in a catabolic state with increased albumin turnover, e.g. in liver disease, fructosamine may be depressed. In these circumstances fructosamine should not be used to monitor glycaemic control.

How should IFCC units be used in clinical practice?

The thermometers displayed here can be used to relate IFCC HbA$_{1c}$ (in mmol/mol) to DCCT results (in percentage) and also to visualise the relationships between an IFCC HbA$_{1c}$ value and a patient's risk of the various complications of diabetes (Figure 13).

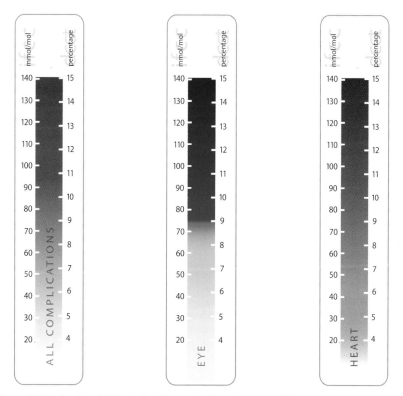

Figure 13 Relationship of IFCC units for HbA$_{1c}$ to risk of complications of diabetes.

Table 3 Glycaemic control of patients with diabetes in Birmingham study ($n = 96$)

Glycaemic control	
IFCC HbA$_{1c}$ (mmol/mol)	60 (53–69)
DCCT HbA$_{1c}$ (%)	7.6 (7.0–8.5)
eAG (mmol/l)	9.5 (8.5–10.9)
RPG (mmol/l)	7.3 (5.0–10.8)
Fructosamine (μmol/l)	310 (268–355)
Other factors	
Haemoglobin (g/dl)	13.9 (12.6–15.2)
Reticulocytes × 10⁹/l ($n = 65$)	45.5 (37.8–64.5)
Serum albumin (g/l)	46 (44–47)
Albumin creatinine ratio (ACR) (g/mol) ($n = 71$)	1.1 (0.7–3.8)
Serum creatinine (μmol/l)	101 (87–113)

The graphs in Figure 14 relate IFCC HbA$_{1c}$ to random plasma glucose (RPG) and fructosamine. They were obtained from a research study performed in Birmingham, UK, where venous blood was collected and sent to the laboratory for plasma glucose measurement. HbA$_{1c}$ was measured by HPLC using a Tosoh G8 analyser with no variant haemoglobin detected. Ninety-six white Caucasian patients (64 males, 29 with type 1 diabetes and the others with type 2 diabetes), attending the diabetes clinic, were aged 61 (51–71) years, with BMI 31.5 (26.8–35.6) kg/m², median (IQ range). No patients had low haemoglobin, reticulocytes outside the reference interval, or proteinuria (Table 3).

Average or mean plasma glucose (eAG) reported for a 24-hour period derived from HbA$_{1c}$ was higher than random plasma glucose measured 2.5 hours after the last meal (the lower quartile 2.0 hours and the upper quartile 3.3 hours).

Weak correlation was shown between RPG and IFCC HbA$_{1c}$ (Pearson correlation coefficient $r = 0.52$), and between RPG and fructosamine, ($r = 0.46$); both $p<0.001$.

What HbA$_{1c}$ values should be expected?

Haemoglobin is glycated in everyone, irrespective of whether they have diabetes or not, because of the glucose circulating around the body. The reference interval (range) for people who do not have diabetes is 20–40 mmol/mol for IFCC HbA$_{1c}$ and 4–6% in DCCT percentages. The current DCCT HbA$_{1c}$ treatment target range for patients with diabetes of 6.5–7.5% is equivalent to IFCC HbA$_{1c}$ 48–59 mmol/mol.

Low levels of HbA$_{1c}$ below the lower end of the reference interval of 20 mmol/mol (DCCT 4%) can be obtained in people with diabetes and coexisting haematological diseases, nutritional deficiencies or metabolic disorders. Whether these low values actually reflect glycaemic control should be verified by reviewing glucose and fructosamine results (if available). Such low results for HbA$_{1c}$, when found in conditions such as anaemia, can be caused by increased red cell turnover, resulting in a shorter time for glycation. Both the haemoglobin level and reticulocyte count should be reviewed in a patient if their HbA$_{1c}$ is inappropriately low.

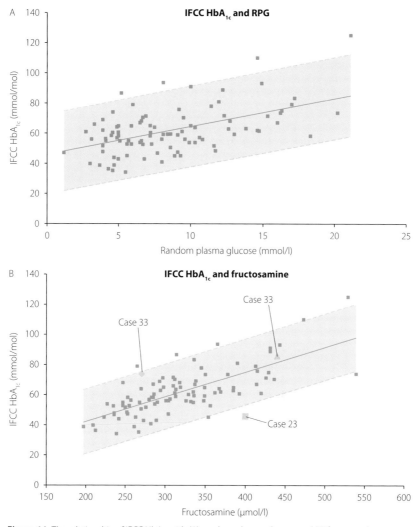

Figure 14 The relationship of IFCC HbA$_{1c}$ with (A) random plasma glucose and (B) fructosamine. ——, linear regression; - - -, 2SD.

High IFCC HbA$_{1c}$ values of 175–195 mmol/mol (DCCT 18%–20%) can be obtained in patients with very poor glycaemic control. Again, glucose or fructosamine should be measured to confirm that the reported HbA$_{1c}$ reflects their glycaemic control. In very rare cases, similarly high HbA$_{1c}$ can be obtained when abnormal haemoglobins such as Camperdown (β104 (G6) arginine → serine) are present, since their separation on HPLC coincides with HbA$_{1c}$. When high HbA$_{1c}$ is not caused by poorly controlled diabetes, concordant plasma glucose and fructosamine values will not be obtained. The Peta Tikva (α110 alanine → aspartic acid) variant elutes at nearly the same position as HbA$_{1c}$ and can cause some elevation of HbA$_{1c}$ when measured by HPLC.

Why is identification of abnormal haemoglobin important?

Not all techniques for measuring HbA$_{1c}$ can detect abnormal haemoglobin. The practice for reporting HbA$_{1c}$ in patients with abnormal haemoglobin varies between laboratories. In heterozygous patients with haemoglobin A as well as abnormal haemoglobin, e.g. AS sickle cell trait, laboratories should either avoid reporting HbA$_{1c}$ or report HbA$_{1c}$ with a caveat that the result cannot be used with targets from clinical guidelines, i.e. it can only be used to assess trends. The reporting of HbA$_{1c}$ in heterozygous patients may be limited to certain variant haemoglobins, e.g. S, C or D as specified by the manufacturers of the particular HbA$_{1c}$ analyser.

There are constraints on issuing HbA$_{1c}$ results in the presence of fetal haemoglobin (HbF) which relate to the technique or analyser used for the measurement of HbA$_{1c}$. When interpreting high HbF, laboratories should be aware that hydroxyurea, sometimes used to treat sickle cell patients, causes an increase in the amount of HbF present in red blood cells. Alternative measures of glycaemic control such as fructosamine or RPG are recommended if HbA$_{1c}$ is not an appropriate measure.

Additional information

IFCC reference method for HbA$_{1c}$

Both the DCCT and the UKPDS included measurement of HbA$_{1c}$ and plasma glucose. For the DCCT, the relationship of HbA$_{1c}$ with mean plasma glucose from self-monitoring of blood glucose (SMBG), seven point profiles, was published and the relationship with FPG was presented for the UKPDS. Several different methods were used to measure glycated haemoglobin in the course of the UKPDS with rigorous comparison of patient data when a new improved method was introduced. The quality of measurements was assessed in both trials, to ensure that values obtained for glycated haemoglobin at the beginning of the trial were equivalent to those obtained at the end. In 1990, the researchers responsible for the UKPDS and DCCT laboratories decided to use the same equipment (the Bio-Rad Diamat HPLC analyser) to measure HbA$_{1c}$, so that changes of 1% HbA$_{1c}$ were equivalent in the two trials.

Why was a reference method required for HbA$_{1c}$?

After the DCCT, a standardisation program, the National Glycohemoglobin Standardization Program (NGSP), was organised in the US to encourage laboratories to report HbA$_{1c}$ values comparable to the DCCT (and later UKPDS). Subsequently all laboratories in the US and UK changed to reporting DCCT HbA$_{1c}$ in percentages.

Since no higher-level reference method was available for HbA$_{1c}$, the IFCC took the lead in establishing one. They synthesised pure HbA$_{1c}$ and non-glycated haemoglobin HbA$_0$, which were measured by mass spectrometry and capillary electrophoresis. Although the IFCC reference method is now the best available for

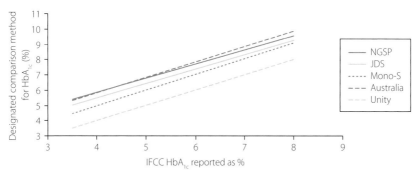

Figure 15 Relationship of IFCC HbA$_{1c}$ with other standardisation programs.

measurement of HbA$_{1c}$, it is too expensive for measuring samples from individual patients. However, this method has been used to calibrate field methods for HbA$_{1c}$ since December 2003 in response to an EC directive requiring that the highest-order method be used for calibration of instrumentation.

HbA$_{1c}$ results for patients' samples obtained from the IFCC reference method were compared with to those from the different standardisation programs used throughout the world: the DCCT from the US, the Mono S from Sweden and the Japanese Diabetes Society (JDS) from Japan (Figure 15).

The IFCC reference method gave HbA$_{1c}$ values that were lower than the DCCT method, as it was more specific for HbA$_{1c}$. However, reporting lower values obtained from the IFCC method could have caused glycaemic control to worsen, because patients might have relaxed their control. It was for this reason the international consensus committee decided in 2007 that reporting of Système Internationale (SI) units for the international reference method, i.e. mmol HbA$_{1c}$/mol unglycated haemoglobin, was preferable to IFCC percentages.

Abnormal haemoglobin

Different haemoglobin variants occur typically in peoples from various parts of the world, with sickle cell haemoglobin prevalent in Africa, India and parts of the Middle East, haemoglobin C in West Africa, and haemoglobin D Punjab in Pakistan (Figure 16). These common haemoglobinopathies, caused by single amino acid substitutions in the β globin chain, affect the structure of haemoglobin and in some cases also the size and shape of red blood cells (Table 4). In the heterozygous state they are relatively benign but in the homozygous state, or combined with another abnormal haemoglobin, can cause serious disease, e.g. sickle cell disease. Genetic abnormalities also cause α and β thalassaemias with decreased production of the respective globin chains. Hundreds of haemoglobin variants are listed on http://globin.cse.psu.edu

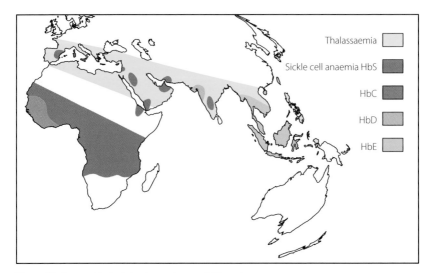

Figure 16 Geographical origin of some haemoglobin variants.

Table 4 Amino acid substitutions in variant haemoglobins.

Hb variant	Amino acid substitution
HbS β6	glutamic acid → valine
HbC β6	glutamic acid → lysine
HbD Punjab β121	glutamic acid → glutamine
HbE β26	glutamic acid → lysine

These geographical patterns are gradually changing, given the increased ease of migration in the 21st century. The prevalence of variant haemoglobins varies across the UK, with higher rates in those parts of the country such as London and the West Midlands with a wide range of ethnic groups.

Data published for the UK neonatal screening program in London and the south-east of England show that haemoglobin AS (57%), AC (14%), AD (8.6%), AE (7.1%) and SS (1.8%) were the most common haemoglobinopathies found in the region. A similar pattern was found in a South Birmingham hospital (unpublished data). If patients with variant haemoglobin identified from the neonatal screening program were to be tagged on hospital IT systems, this would be beneficial if they were to develop diabetes in later life. It is important to recognise whether patients have variant haemoglobin, as not enough is known about the glycation of variant haemoglobin.

Measurement of HbA$_{1c}$

High performance liquid chromatography (HPLC)

Haemoglobins are separated from each other according to their charge, with the output from the analyser displayed as peaks indicating the presence of glycated, fetal or abnormal haemoglobins. These chromatograms are inspected to determine the value of HbA$_{1c}$ and whether a patient has abnormal haemoglobin/s or raised fetal haemoglobin (HbF >5%) (Figure 17). HbA$_{1c}$ cannot be reported if a patient is homozygous for abnormal haemoglobin (e.g. SS sickle cell anaemia) or heterozygous for two abnormal haemoglobins (e.g. SC) as no haemoglobin A is

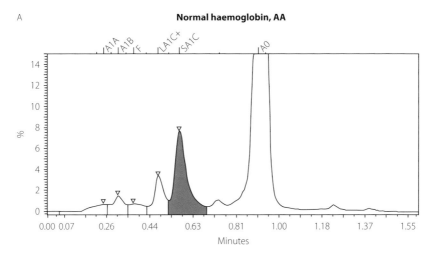

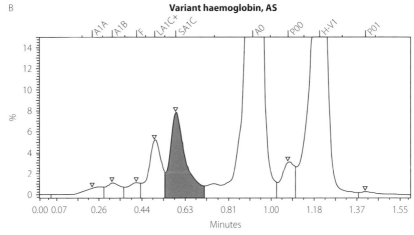

Figure 17 Chromatograms from TOSOH G8 HPLC analyser, for normal and variant haemoglobins (blue panel indicates HbA$_{1c}$).

Measurement of HbA$_{1c}$

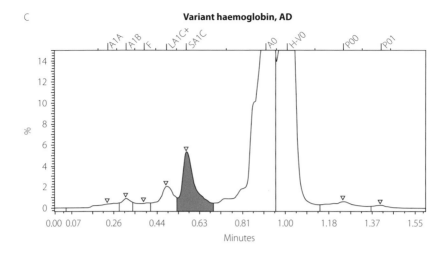

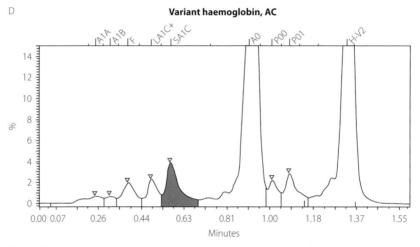

Figure 17 (*Continued*)

present. HPLC analysers are mainly situated in hospitals rather than GP clinics because of their cost and the expertise required to interpret their output. Users of a particular HPLC analyser should ask the manufacturer whether HbA$_{1c}$ can be reported in the presence of different variant haemoglobin or fetal haemoglobin.

Immunochemistry

HbA$_{1c}$ can be measured using immunochemistry on automated laboratory analysers, smaller point-of-care analysers such as the DCA 2000, and disposable cartridges, e.g. Metrika. The technique uses antibodies to measure HbA$_{1c}$ with

Measurement of HbA$_{1c}$

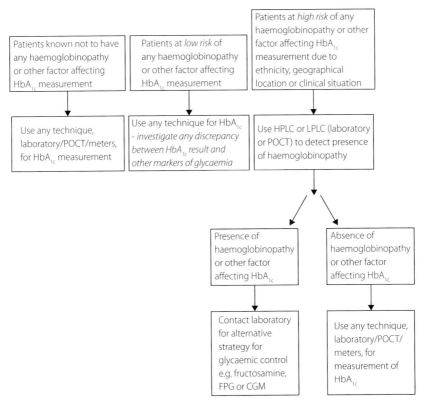

Figure 18 Selection of appropriate method for measurement of HbA₁c.

the specificity of the antibody determining whether or not glycated variant hae-moglobins are recognised in addition to normal haemoglobin. It is advisable to contact manufacturers for more information on measurement of HbA₁c when ab-normal haemoglobin is present especially fetal haemoglobin. Information may be not always be available for rarer variant haemoglobins and their effects on specific analytical systems.

Affinity chromatography
This type of chromatography relies on the differential binding of glycated proteins to a boronate column, rather than on differences in charge. The HbA₁c values re-ported will include any glycated abnormal haemoglobins present as well as normal glycated haemoglobin. However, it is not known if normal and variant haemo-globins bind glucose at the same rate.

The flow sheet presented in Figure 18 describes how to select an appropriate method for HbA₁c measurement for different patients. It should be noted that

Measurement of HbA₁c

	n	Mean	SD	CV(%)
Derived	275	53.4	1.7	3.2
Axis Shield Afinion	4	50.0		
Bayer DCA 2000	48	54.4	1.7	3.1
Beckman Synchron/LX	2	52.0		
BioRad D-10	5	54.0	3.0	5.5
BioRad Variant (II)	24	53.3	2.8	5.3
Menarini HA 8140	3	54.0		
Menarini HA 8160	89	52.7	1.1	2.1
Primus	8	52.5	2.7	5.1
Siemens DCA Vantage [5TE8]	14	53.8	1.9	3.5
Tosoh G7	42	53.9	0.8	1.5
Tosoh G8 [5TO8]	28	54.7	1.2	2.2

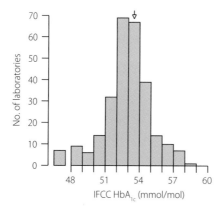

Your result	54
Target value (GLTM)	53.4
Your specimen:	
%bias	+1.1
transformed bias	0
Accuracy Index	0
Secondary IFCC value	54.4
DCCT comp. value	7.13
ALTM (for information only)	53.43

Figure 19 Variation in HbA$_{1c}$ results for the same sample, measured by different methods.

Measurement of HbA$_{1c}$

small differences in HbA$_{1c}$ may result from use of different analysers, possibly related to the particular technique/equipment used and the calibration (Figure 19). The extract from a quality assurance scheme subscribed to by laboratories shows how results for the same blood sample can vary when measured by different methods and in different places.

Measurement of glucose

Most laboratory protocols recommend particular tubes (usually containing fluoride oxalate as a preservative) for collection of blood (Figure 20). These are sent to the laboratory and centrifuged on receipt to separate red blood cells from the liquid known as plasma, used for measurement.

Plasma glucose should ideally be measured within 30 minutes of collection of blood (or centrifuged with the plasma stored for analysis later). It is rarely possible to analyse blood specimens within this timeframe when transporting samples to the laboratory from general practice, a ward or an outpatient clinic. Despite the use of inhibitors of glucose metabolism like fluoride oxalate, glucose metabolism in red blood cells is not halted immediately after collection, and delays lead to a lowering of glucose values by about 0.5 to 1.0 mmol/l.

Venous plasma glucose

Blood samples obtained from a patient's vein in a hospital ward or GP clinic are sent to a laboratory for measurement of venous plasma glucose. The blood is centrifuged before being placed on a large, high volume, automated analyser.

Capillary plasma glucose or blood glucose

Fingers can be pricked with a lancet and capillary glucose measured in the resulting drop of blood on blood glucose meters calibrated to either plasma or blood. Some patients with diabetes carry out self-monitoring of blood glucose (SMBG) using glucose meters. Their glucose results and the timing can be stored in the meter memory and downloaded remotely to a patient's computer or by their healthcare team.

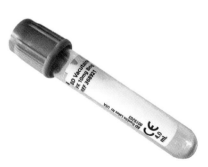

Figure 20 Tube for collection of blood for measurement of plasma glucose in the laboratory.

Measurement of glucose

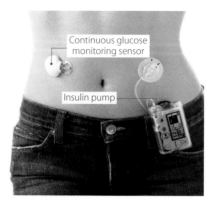

Figure 21 Continuous glucose monitoring sensor (left) and an insulin pump (right).

On hospital wards or in outpatient clinics, blood glucose meters may be used to measure glucose, with very high or low values confirmed in the laboratory. Most meters used in the UK are calibrated to report values corresponding to plasma, but some may still be calibrated for blood. This can cause confusion to both patients and health care professionals. Results for glucose measured in whole blood are lower than from plasma, and should be multiplied by a factor of 1.1 to obtain equivalent plasma values. Manufacturers' instruction leaflets and websites should be consulted to determine whether a particular meter reports glucose results in relation to blood or plasma, as it is vital to compare like with like when setting targets or following clinical guidelines.

Average or mean plasma glucose over 24 hours
Newer, continuous blood glucose monitoring devices use a sensor that is placed in the abdomen to monitor glucose in the interstitial fluid (that bathes cells) continuously over the course of 24 hours, for a period up to 6 days (Figure 21). They are usually calibrated to report plasma equivalents, i.e. mean or average plasma glucose. These devices were used in the ADAG study and are located in the body in a similar place to insulin pumps.

Two-hour glucose from OGTT
In some circumstances, e.g. for diagnosis of IGT or diabetes, or during pregnancy, or after a coronary event, a patient may be requested to attend a clinic or laboratory for an OGTT. Following measurement of fasting plasma glucose, the patient drinks a glucose load (usually equivalent to 75g of anhydrous glucose), and plasma glucose is measured after two hours (2 hour plasma glucose, 2hPG). Although most OGTT glucose results are reported as plasma glucose, in a few hospitals an analyser such as a Yellow Springs Instrument (YSI) may be used to determine blood glucose.

Measurement of glucose

References

American Diabetes Association. Diagnosis and classification of diabetes mellitus. Clinical Practice Recommendations 2008: Position Statement. *Diabetes Care* 2008;**31:**S55–S60.

Cohen RM, Franco RS, Khera PK, Smith EP, Lindsell CJ, Ciraolo PJ *et al.* Red cell life span heterogeneity in hematologically normal people is sufficient to alter HbA$_{1c}$. *Blood* 2008;**112:**4284–91.

DCCT Study Group. The effect of intensive treatment of diabetes on the development and progression of long-term complications of insulin-dependent diabetes mellitus; the Diabetes Control and Complications Trial. *N Engl J Med* 1993;**329:**977–86.

Hoelzel W, Weykamp C, Jeppson J-O, Miedema K, Barr JR, Goodall I *et al.* IFCC reference system for measurement of haemoglobin A$_{1c}$ in human blood and the national standardization schemes in the United States, Japan, and Sweden: a method-comparison study. *Clin Chem* 2004;**50:**166–74.

IDF Clinical Guidelines Task Force. Global Guidelines for Type 2 Diabetes. *Brussels: International Diabetic Federation* 2005;26–8.

Manley S. Haemoglobin A$_{1c}$ – a marker for complications of type 2 diabetes: the experience from the UK Prospective Diabetes Study (UKPDS). *Clin Chem Lab Med* 2003;**41:**1182–90.

Manley SE. Estimated average glucose derived from HbA$_{1c}$ (eAG): report from European Association for the Study of Diabetes (EASD), Amsterdam 2007. *Diabet Med* 2008;**25:**126–8.

Manley SE, Cull CA, Holman RR. Relationship of HbA$_{1c}$ to fasting plasma glucose in patients with Type 2 diabetes in the UKPDS randomised to and treated with diet or oral agents. *Diabetes* 2000;**49:**A180, 742-P.

Manley SE, Gomes AN, McKnight JA, Ritchie SA, Geddes J, Stratton IM *et al.* When fructosamine results for patients do not reflect glycaemic control indicated by other markers. *Diabet Med* 2009;**26** Suppl 1:P390.

Manley S, John WG, Marshall S. Introduction of IFCC reference method for calibration of HbA$_{1c}$: implications for clinical care. *Diabet Med* 2004;**21:**673–6.

Manley SE, Moore S, Smith JM, Cramb R. When HbA$_{1c}$ for a patient does not reflect glycaemic control indicated by plasma glucose monitoring. *Diabet Med* 2008;**25:**P256.

Manley SE, Round RA, Smith JM. Calibration of HbA$_{1c}$ and its measurement in the presence of variant haemoglobins: report on questionnaire to manufacturers. *Ann Clin Biochem* 2006;**43:**135–45.

Manley SE, Sikaris KA, Lu ZX, Nightingale PG, Stratton IM, Round RA *et al.* Validation of an algorithm combining haemoglobin A$_{1c}$ and fasting plasma glucose for diagnosis of diabetes mellitus in UK and Australian populations *Diabet Med* 2009;**26:**115–21.

Manley SE, Stratton IM, Clark PM, Luzio SD. Comparison of 11 human insulin assays: implications for clinical investigation and research. *Clin Chem* 2007;**53:**922–32.

Nathan DM, Kuenne J, Borg R, Zheng H, Schoenfeld D, Heine RJ. Translating the A$_{1c}$ assay into estimated average glucose values. *Diabetes Care* 2008;**31:**1473–9.

NICE. Management of Blood Glucose. NICE Clinical Guideline G. London: National Institute for Clinical Excellence 2008. Available at http://www.nice.org.uk

Rohlfing CL, Wiedmeyer H-M, Little RR, England JD, Tennill A, Goldstein DE. Defining the relationship between plasma glucose and HbA$_{1c}$ analysis of glucose profiles and HbA$_{1c}$ in the Diabetes Control and Complications Trial. *Diabetes Care* 2002;**25:**275–8.

UK Prospective Diabetes Study Group. UKPDS XI: Biochemical risk factors in Type 2 diabetic patients at diagnosis compared with age-matched normal subjects. *Diabet Med* 1994;**11**:534–44.

UK Prospective Diabetes Study Group. UKPDS 33: Intensive blood-glucose control with sulphonylureas or insulin compared with conventional treatment and risk of complications in patients with type 2 diabetes. *Lancet* 1998;**352**:837–53.

UK Prospective Diabetes Study Group. UKPDS 35: Association of glycaemia with macrovascular and microvascular complications of type 2 diabetes: prospective observational study. *BMJ* 2000;**321**:405–12.

WHO Study Group on Diabetes Mellitus. Diabetes Mellitus: Report of a WHO study group. WHO technical report series no. 727. Geneva: World Health Organization, 1985.

Case studies

Colour key to case studies

The headings and appropriate NICE Guidelines for the case studies are colour-coded as follows:

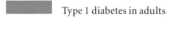 Type 1 diabetes in adults

Type 1 diabetes in children and young people

Type 2 diabetes

Diabetes in pregnancy

The icon on each case study identifies the patient group:

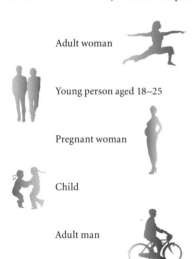

Adult woman

Young person aged 18–25

Pregnant woman

Child

Adult man

1: Diagnosis and early management of type 1 diabetes in a young child

Julie A. Edge, Consultant in Paediatric Diabetes, Oxford, UK

Background

A four-year-old child was seen by her GP with a two-week history of polyuria and polydipsia, as well as bedwetting at night. Capillary blood glucose at the time was 23.2 mmol/l. The GP diagnosed diabetes and referred the girl on the same day to the children's diabetes team at the local hospital. On admission the child was clinically well, a little dry but eating and drinking with no nausea or vomiting. Her parents felt that she had lost a little weight, therefore no intravenous fluid or insulin was required. A clinical diagnosis of type 1 diabetes was made.

Treatment plan

IFCC 91 ≡ DCCT 10.5%

Baseline tests taken at the time later found an IFCC HbA$_{1c}$ level of 91 mmol/mol, and positive islet-cell antibodies, confirming type 1 diabetes. She was started on subcutaneous insulin in a multiple injection regimen, using a preprandial rapid-acting analogue with once-daily basal long-acting analogue, given in the morning because of her age. Her parents were taught carbohydrate counting within the first week.

Follow-up

For the first two weeks on this regimen, the child's appetite was ravenous but blood glucose levels were all within the normal range (4–7 mmol/l) with an insulin dose of around 0.7 units/kg/day. By two months the dose had fallen to 0.3 units/kg/day and the child's appetite had returned to normal. IFCC

IFCC 71 ≡ DCCT 8.6%

HbA$_{1c}$ had fallen to 71 mmol/mol.

IFCC 46 ≡ DCCT 6.4%

Three months after diagnosis, IFCC HbA$_{1c}$ was down to 46 mmol/mol and the family were beginning to become accustomed to the new regimen. One year after diagnosis, her IFCC HbA$_{1c}$ remained within the target range at

IFCC 52 ≡ DCCT 6.9%

52 mmol/mol. The teachers and teaching assistants at her new school had been taught how to test blood glucose levels and to administer her lunchtime insulin dose.

NICE Guidelines: Type 1 diabetes in children and young people
HbA$_{1c}$ target: IFCC <59 mmol/mol ≡ <7.5%

2: Management of an elderly patient, housebound and living alone
Chris Cottrell and Helen Green, Diabetes Specialist Nurses, Llanelli, Wales, UK

Background
An 89-year-old man with type 2 diabetes, diagnosed in 1992, had a history of hypertension and chronic renal disease stage 4 (estimated glomerular filtration rate 27ml/min/1.73m^2). He lived alone in a bungalow. With IFCC HbA$_{1c}$ at 65 mmol/mol, he was started on a once daily long acting insulin analogue. He was also taking aspirin 75 mg daily; bisoprolol 2.5 mg daily; quinine 200 mg at night; furosemide 80 mg daily; simvastatin 20 mg at night. His lipid profile was within the target range. Blood pressure was 138/50 mmHg and he was asymptomatic.

IFCC 65 ≡ DCCT 8.1%

The patient was referred to the diabetes nurse within the chronic disease management team about 12 months after starting insulin, because his daughter reported that her father was afraid of having a hypoglycaemic attack and was taking a high-calorie drink during the day following his insulin injection. He may have been having hypoglycaemic episodes due to a cumulative effect of insulin and renal disease. IFCC HbA$_{1c}$ was down to 52 mmol/mol.

IFCC 52 ≡ DCCT 6.9%

Treatment plan
The main aim was to prevent hypoglycaemia, falls and reduce his anxiety level. Frequent visits, carers in attendance twice daily and an education plan were implemented. A 'lifeline' system was introduced to ensure safety, and home modifications made to maintain his safety and independence. In view of his chronic renal disease, it was not appropriate to start him on ACE/ARB therapy. Because of this, IFCC HbA$_{1c}$ of 52 mmol/mol was defined as too low and his insulin regimen was reduced accordingly.

IFCC 52 ≡ DCCT 6.9%

Follow-up
The patient was housebound, but able to self-administer his insulin and medication. He had no further hypoglycaemic episodes. IFCC HbA$_{1c}$ was 65 mmol/mol with no symptoms of hyperglycaemia. He had regular follow-up visits by the diabetes nurse and a contact number for advice. He remained happy because his main wish was to remain in his own home.

IFCC 65 ≡ DCCT 8.1%

NICE Guidelines: Type 2 diabetes
HbA$_{1c}$ targets: IFCC 48 mmol/mol ≡ 6.5% to IFCC 59 mmol/mol ≡ 7.5%

3: Gestational diabetes

Jonathan Webber, Consultant Physician, Birmingham, UK

Background

A 29-year-old obese Asian woman (BMI 28 kg/m²), with a family history of type 2 diabetes became pregnant. At 26 weeks' gestation her fasting whole blood glucose was 7.3 mmol/l and two-hour value at OGTT 11.4 mmol/l (GDM≥7.8 mmol/l). She was referred to the antenatal diabetes clinic, where her initial IFCC HbA₁c at diagnosis of gestational diabetes was 59 mmol/mol. The raised HbA₁c at diagnosis suggested she may have had impaired glucose tolerance or diabetes prior to pregnancy.

IFCC 59 ≡ DCCT 7.5%

Treatment plan

After assessment by a diabetologist and obstetrician, she was given dietetic and lifestyle advice by a dietician. She was also given a glucose meter and shown how to use it. Targets were given for fasting and pre-meal glucose (between 3.5 and 5.9 mmol/l) and for less than 7.8 mmol/l one hour after meals.

At 28 weeks' gestation, most of her post-meal glucose values were above 10.0 mmol/l and her fasting and pre-meal glucose values were between 6.0 and 7.0 mmol/l. The growth scan showed an increased abdominal circumference and a fetal weight above the 90th centile. She was started on short-acting insulin three times a day with meals, and an isophane insulin before going to bed.

Over the next ten weeks her insulin doses were regularly monitored and adjusted. Subsequent scans showed growth above the 90th centile. Labour was induced between 38 and 39 weeks, but she required a Caesarean section and delivered a boy of 4.5 kg. Insulin treatment was stopped immediately after delivery.

Follow-up

Six weeks after the birth her fasting glucose was 6.6 mmol/l with 10.3 mmol/l after two hours. She was told she had impaired glucose tolerance. IFCC HbA₁c was 42 mmol/mol. She was discharged to the care of her GP, with further advice on dietary and lifestyle changes to reduce her high risk of subsequent type 2 diabetes. Annual fasting glucose testing was recommended. If planning further pregnancies she should be seen in the pre-conception diabetes clinic, and restart home blood glucose monitoring.

IFCC 42 ≡ DCCT 6.0%

NICE Guidelines: Diabetes in pregnancy
HbA₁c target prepregnancy*: IFCC <43 mmol/mol ≡ <6.1%
*(if safely achievable)

4: Weight loss and improved glycaemic control
Pamela Dyson, Dietician, Oxford, UK

Background
A 56-year-old woman weighing 89.3 kg (BMI 36.5 kg/m^2), who had been diagnosed four years previously with type 2 diabetes was referred to a diabetes
specialist dietician for lifestyle advice and weight loss. At diagnosis, she had
been prescribed metformin 500 mg once daily, and after three months her
IFCC HbA$_{1c}$ values decreased from 69 to 59 mmol/mol. Over the next four   IFCC 69 ≡ DCCT 8.5%
years, metformin doses had been titrated up and gliclazide added, until she   IFCC 59 ≡ DCCT 7.5%
was taking maximum dose of both agents. At her latest appointment, glycae-
mic control was suboptimal with IFCC HbA$_{1c}$ value of 77 mmol/mol. It was   IFCC 77 ≡ DCCT 9.2%
recommended that she start insulin therapy, but she was very resistant to
this idea and insisted that she have a trial of weight loss for 3 months before
insulin was initiated.

Treatment plan
Despite receiving dietary advice at diagnosis, she freely admitted that she
had never attempted to change her dietary intake or to lose weight. During
consultation, she identified that she consumed a high fat diet with frequent
snacks and that she had a sedentary lifestyle. She decided that she would opt
for a reduced fat, reduced sugar diet, avoid snacks and purchase a pedometer
with the aim of walking 10 000 steps each day. Her target IFCC HbA$_{1c}$ was
<53 mmol/mol.   IFCC 53 ≡ DCCT 7.0%

Follow-up
Three months after changing her lifestyle by increasing physical activity and
reducing dietary intake, she had reduced her weight by 7.4 kg (8.2%), her
IFCC HbA$_{1c}$ had decreased to 57 mmol/mol and she had halved her gliclazide   IFCC 57 ≡ DCCT 7.4%
dose to 80 mg twice daily. Over the next year, she continued to lose weight
and maintained her IFCC HbA$_{1c}$ levels with values of 53 and 55 mmol/mol.   IFCC 53 ≡ DCCT 7.0%
She now accepts that although she has been able to improve her glycaemic   IFCC 55 ≡ DCCT 7.2%
control by lifestyle change, she will probably need insulin therapy at some
time in the future.

NICE Guidelines: Type 2 diabetes
HbA$_{1c}$ targets: IFCC 48 mmol/mol ≡ 6.5% to IFCC 59 mmol/mol ≡ 7.5%

5: Type 2 diabetes in a child

Timothy G. Barrett, Professor of Paediatric Endocrinology, Birmingham, UK

Background

An eight-year-old girl was diagnosed in 2003 with type 2 diabetes on the basis of fasting glucose of 11 mmol/l and two-hour glucose of 17.8 mmol/l. She was obese from the age of six years and developed acanthosis nigricans in her neck and limb flexures. By the time of the glucose tolerance test she had developed thirst and was waking at night for a drink. She had primary nocturnal enuresis and some accidents during the day. Both her parents were well but both maternal grandparents had diabetes. Her ethnic origin was from India via East Africa. Her fasting insulin was 281 pmol/l (raised) and IFCC HbA$_{1c}$ 68 mmol/mol. Her GAD and islet cell antibodies were negative. She weighed 60 kg (BMI above 99.6th centile for age).

IFCC 68 ≡ DCCT 8.4%

Treatment plan

In view of her obesity, she was given an intensive lifestyle education programme, and started on metformin. Initially her IFCC HbA$_{1c}$ fell to 53, but as lifestyle began to revert, it increased to 68 mmol/mol and metformin was increased to 500 mg, 12-hourly. She was screened for retinopathy, microalbuminuria, liver function and fasting lipids (all normal). A random glucose check on her mother gave a result of 11.2 mmol/l; so she was referred to the adult diabetes team, although very reluctant to acknowledge that she also had diabetes.

IFCC 53 ≡ DCCT 7.0%
IFCC 68 ≡ DCCT 8.4%

Follow-up

The daughter's IFCC HbA$_{1c}$ increased to 89 mmol/mol in 2005, at which point insulin was added at 0.5 units/kg/day. Her IFCC HbA$_{1c}$ improved to 76 mmol/mol initially, but within six months was back up to 89 mmol/mol and her weight was 80.6 kg. Over the next six months she stopped taking insulin; IFCC HbA$_{1c}$ increased to 112 mmol/mol and she lost 4 kg in weight. She was admitted to the ward for continuous intravenous insulin infusion and recalculation of her insulin requirements, and with play therapy support she overcame her fear of injections. Her current IFCC HbA$_{1c}$ is 74 mmol/mol. CSII pump therapy is recommended.

IFCC 89 ≡ DCCT 10.3%

IFCC 76 ≡ DCCT 9.1%
IFCC 89 ≡ DCCT 10.3%
IFCC 112 ≡ DCCT 12.4%

IFCC 74 ≡ DCCT 8.9%

NICE Guidelines: Type 2 diabetes
HbA$_{1c}$ targets: IFCC 48 mmol/mol ≡ 6.5% to IFCC 59 mmol/mol ≡ 7.5%

6: Weight reduction

G. Pooler R. Archbold, Ailish G. Nugent and R. Welby Henry, Consultant Chemical Pathologist (GPRA), Consultant Physicians (AGN, RWH), Belfast, Northern Ireland, UK

Background

This lady had been diagnosed with type 2 diabetes in 2001 at the age of 45 years. She had no symptoms related to diabetes, but weighed 144.5 kg (BMI 50.7 kg/m^2). Initially, fasting venous glucose was 11.1 mmol/l, IFCC HbA$_{1c}$ 73 mmol/mol, creatinine 84 µmol/l, cholesterol 7.5 mmol/l, triglycerides 2.21 mmol/l, HDL-cholesterol 0.8 mmol/l; thyroid function normal. Blood pressure was normal, and she did not smoke cigarettes or drink alcohol.

IFCC 73 ≡ DCCT 8.8%

Treatment plan

She was started on metformin 500 mg three times daily and simvastatin 40 mg daily, and given close dietetic support with the aim of weight reduction (no target specified) and achievement of IFCC HbA$_{1c}$ 53 mmol/mol.

IFCC 53 ≡ DCCT 7.0%

Follow-up

Initial weight loss led to a progressive fall in HbA$_{1c}$ and by November 2005 weight had leveled off at 125 kg (BMI 43.8 kg/m^2) and IFCC HbA$_{1c}$ 51 mmol/mol. Thereafter, although her weight remained steady, HbA$_{1c}$ started to rise slowly, even with metformin increased to 1000 mg twice daily. By April 2008 her IFCC HbA$_{1c}$ was 67 mmol/mol. At this stage subcutaneous exenatide 5 mg twice daily was added until June 2008, then rising to 10 mg twice daily. The lady's weight fell steadily and by April 2009 was 102 kg (BMI 35.9 kg/m^2), with IFCC HbA$_{1c}$ 38 mmol/mol.

IFCC 51 ≡ DCCT 6.8%

IFCC 67 ≡ DCCT 8.3%

IFCC 38 ≡ DCCT 5.6%

The patient has suffered from nausea with the exenatide but is keen to persist with this treatment. The dose has now been cut back to 5 mg subcutaneously twice daily to try to minimise any risk of hypoglycaemia, and close monitoring will continue. Serum lipids are now controlled with rosuvastatin 20 mg daily.

NICE Guidelines: Type 2 diabetes
HbA$_{1c}$ targets: IFCC 48 mmol/mol ≡ 6.5% to IFCC 59 mmol/mol ≡ 7.5%

7: Improved glycaemic control

Steven Creely, Specialist Registrar in Diabetes and Endocrinology,
Birmingham, UK

Background

A 58-year-old man was diagnosed in 2003 with type 2 diabetes on the basis
of two fasting plasma glucose results over 7 mmol/l. He had no osmotic
symptoms of diabetes (excessive urination, thirst), but was lethargic and
had a BMI of 33 kg/m². He had a strong family history of diabetes, as one
brother and his mother had developed diabetes in their 50s and 60s. He had
a history of hypertension treated with atenolol 50 mg, but his lipid profile
had not been assessed. He smoked 15 cigarettes a day and drank 38 units of
alcohol in a week. At diagnosis, his glycaemic control was suboptimal with

IFCC 89 ≡ DCCT 10.3%

IFCC HbA$_{1c}$ 89 mmol/mol. His total cholesterol was 5.4 mmol/l with HDL
0.9 mmol/l and triglycerides 2.3 mmol/l, and baseline creatinine 96 μmol/l.

Treatment plan

In view of his obesity and hyperglycaemia, appropriate first-line glucose-
lowering therapy would be metformin titrated to maximum treatment effect,

IFCC 53 ≡ DCCT 7.0%

with a target of 53 mmol/mol for IFCC HbA$_{1c}$. Treatment with simvastatin
40 mg should be initiated. As atenolol, his antihypertensive medication, is no
longer considered appropriate within NICE/BHS ACD guidelines, an ACE
inhibitor should be considered for first-line treatment. In addition, advice
should be offered on smoking cessation, reduction in alcohol consumption,
weight loss and diet.

Follow-up

The patient was counselled with lifestyle and dietary advice and started on
metformin 500 mg once daily, which was then titrated to 500 mg three times

IFCC 68 ≡ DCCT 8.4%
IFCC 71 ≡ DCCT 8.6%
IFCC 76 ≡ DCCT 9.1%
IFCC 74 ≡ DCCT 8.9%
IFCC 63 ≡ DCCT 7.9%
IFCC 53 ≡ DCCT 7.0%
IFCC 64 ≡ DCCT 8.0%

daily within two months. His IFCC HbA$_{1c}$ five months after diagnosis was
68, and subsequently over the next year 71, 76 and 74 mmol/mol. The GP
referred the patient to hospital diabetes services. After outpatient review, he
was started on 30/70 mixed insulin, 16 units twice daily and his antihypertensive medication optimised. His IFCC HbA$_{1c}$ at follow-up after 4 months
was 63 mmol/mol. Regular hospital follow-up was continued and his IFCC
HbA$_{1c}$ remained between IFCC 53 and 64 mmol/mol.

NICE Guidelines: Type 2 diabetes
HbA$_{1c}$ targets: IFCC 48 mmol/mol ≡ 6.5% to IFCC 59 mmol/mol ≡ 7.5%

8: Risk of hypoglycaemia in a patient in a unit for the elderly mentally ill in a nursing home

Chris Cottrell and Helen Green, Diabetes Specialist Nurses, Llanelli, Wales, UK

Background

A 72-year-old man with dementia and type 2 diabetes (diagnosed in 1982), hypertension and retinopathy was referred for annual review to the diabetes nurse in the chronic disease management team. He was living in a unit for the elderly mentally ill in a private nursing home. Staff at the home advised that he was aggressive and that he would not allow an examination to be conducted.

His blood glucose levels were determined daily within the home, and his fasting blood glucose levels were all <4.0 mmol/l. He was usually in a hypoglycaemic state on waking. He was unable to converse appropriately and was therefore unable to convey his symptoms without being aggressive, which was attributed to his mental state. His IFCC HbA$_{1c}$ was 46 mmol/mol. He was being treated with gliclazide 80 mg daily.

IFCC 46 ≡ DCCT 6.4%

Treatment plan

Gliclazide was stopped. His creatinine level was 233 μmol/l (normal range 62–106 μmol/l). NICE guidelines suggest metformin should not be initiated if creatinine level is above 150 μmol/l, therefore metformin would have been inappropriate to use. He was a thin gentleman, weighing 58 kg with BMI 21.5 kg/m^2. The main treatment aim was to prevent hypoglycaemia.

An education programme was started for all staff within the nursing home. It covered the nature of diabetes and its complications, causes, symptoms of hypoglycaemia and hyperglycaemia and their treatment, and blood glucose monitoring.

Follow-up

When reviewed one month later, nursing home staff reported that he was now very pleasant and approachable, and was agreeable to interventions since stopping gliclazide. There was no further history of hypoglycaemia. At his diabetes annual review, which included a foot examination, his IFCC HbA$_{1c}$ was 44 mmol/mol. There has been no further history of hypoglycaemia and he continues to be pleasant and manageable within the home environment. He is followed up annually and as required by the chronic disease management team.

IFCC 44 ≡ DCCT 6.2%

NICE Guidelines: Type 2 diabetes
HbA$_{1c}$ targets: IFCC 48 mmol/mol ≡ 6.5% to IFCC 59 mmol/mol ≡ 7.5%

9: Structured education for type 1 diabetes
Pamela Dyson, Dietician, Oxford, UK

Background
A 32-year-old man was referred for a structured education programme to develop skills for carbohydrate counting and insulin adjustment. He had been diagnosed with type 1 diabetes when aged 12 and had recently expressed concern about his glycaemic control, following routine eye screening which had identified background retinopathy. His recent IFCC HbA$_{1c}$ value was 70 mmol/mol but he had seen a report on the Diabetes UK website recommending a target IFCC HbA$_{1c}$ of 48 mmol/mol. In the past, he had found that reducing his blood glucose levels resulted in increased hypoglycaemia. His current insulin regimen was: long-acting insulin 26 units once daily and insulin aspart 8–10 units three times daily with meals.

IFCC 70 ≡ DCCT 8.6%
IFCC 48 ≡ DCCT 6.5%

Treatment plan
He took part in a group education programme designed for people with type 1 diabetes. The course consisted of 15 hours' education over four weeks and was based upon adult learning theories. The course was facilitated jointly by a diabetes specialist nurse and a diabetes specialist dietician. In addition to carbohydrate counting and insulin adjustment, it addressed management of hypoglycaemia, hyperglycaemia, exercise, alcohol and illness. At the end of the course, his basal insulin remained at 26 units and he adopted the regimen of injecting 1 unit of insulin aspart for every 10 g carbohydrate eaten. As hypoglycaemia was of concern, he decided to aim for a target IFCC HbA$_{1c}$ of 53 mmol/mol.

IFCC 53 ≡ DCCT 7.0%

Follow-up
Six months after completing the course, his glycaemic control had improved and his IFCC HbA$_{1c}$ was 55 mmol/mol. In the two years following the course, he has had his HbA$_{1c}$ measured at six-monthly intervals and, by adopting the approach of carbohydrate counting and insulin adjustment, has maintained his IFCC HbA$_{1c}$ at just above his target with values between 54 and 57 mmol/mol, without significant increase in hypoglycaemia.

IFCC 55 ≡ DCCT 7.2%

IFCC 54 ≡ DCCT 7.1%
IFCC 57 ≡ DCCT 7.4%

NICE Guidelines: Type 1 diabetes in adults
HbA$_{1c}$ targets: IFCC 48 mmol/mol ≡ 6.5% to IFCC 59 mmol/mol ≡ 7.5%

10: Woman with family history of raised cholesterol and diabetes

Robert Cramb, Consultant Chemical Pathologist, Birmingham, UK

Background

A 60-year-old woman was referred to the lipid clinic for review. She had been diagnosed with hypertension ten years previously and was prescribed a diuretic, bendroflumethiazide 2.5 mg once daily, and an ACE inhibitor to control her blood pressure, lisinopril 20 mg once daily. She reported an episode of chest pain that was investigated. She was discovered to have an aortic murmur but an exercise electrocardiogram, ECG, and concurrent echocardiogram showed no abnormalities. There was a family history of increased cholesterol but no history of early heart disease. Her 72-year-old sister was known to be hypertensive and her 70-year-old brother had been diagnosed with diabetes.

Treatment plan

Serum cholesterol measurement was requested by the GP practice and was 7.2 mmol/l at presentation. Her GP commenced statin treatment, simvastatin (40 mg once daily) but referred her to the lipid clinic for advice. After the use of simvastatin for at least 6 weeks, her total cholesterol was reviewed in the Lipid Clinic and showed a decrease of 21%, to 5.7 mmol/l. As this decrease in cholesterol was smaller than expected, other relevant parameters were reviewed. Her fasting plasma glucose concentration was found to be 7.9 mmol/l, indicating diabetes, and her IFCC HbA$_{1c}$ was 63 mmol/mol.

IFCC 63 ≡ DCCT 7.9%

Follow-up

The patient was prescribed metformin at 500 mg twice daily. After a further two months with no additional lipid-lowering therapy, her total cholesterol concentration was reduced to 3.4 mmol/l and her IFCC HbA$_{1c}$ to 53 mmol/mol.

IFCC 53 ≡ DCCT 7.0%

NICE Guidelines: Type 2 diabetes
HbA$_{1c}$ targets: IFCC 48 mmol/mol ≡ 6.5% to IFCC 59 mmol/mol ≡ 7.5%

11: Type 1 diabetes in a child

Timothy G. Barrett, Professor of Paediatric Endocrinology, Birmingham, UK

Background

A nine-year-old boy with a two-day history of polydipsia and polyuria was referred to the emergency department by his GP. He had weight loss over the past two to three weeks, and had been feeling tired for two weeks. He had no family history of diabetes. His capillary glucose was 27.9 mmol/l with ketonuria, but he was not acidotic. He was started on multiple daily insulin injections, and managed at home with nurse visits at injection times for the first three to five days. His IFCC HbA$_{1c}$ at diagnosis was 95 mmol/mol. He was a very sporty lad, participating in football and ballet.

IFCC 95 ≡ DCCT 10.8%

Treatment plan

He was started on insulin 0.5 units/kg/day, consisting of insulin aspart with meals and insulin glargine 6 units in the evening. He and his family started carbohydrate counting within three days, initially using one unit of insulin aspart for every 20 g carbohydrate at each meal. Within two months his IFCC HbA$_{1c}$ fell to 65 mmol/mol, then to 54 mmol/mol by five months after diagnosis. His insulin requirements remained low, indicating he was in the honeymoon period. He was taught to use correction boluses of one unit of insulin to bring the glucose down by 5 mmol/l, to an initial target of 7.5 mmol/l.

IFCC 65 ≡ DCCT 8.1%
IFCC 54 ≡ DCCT 7.1%

Follow-up

IFCC 63 ≡ DCCT 7.9%

By 11 months after diagnosis, his IFCC HbA$_{1c}$ had increased to 63 mmol/mol with capillary glucose results rising during the day to 10 mmol/l. His insulin:carbohydrate ratio was increased and additional insulin glargine given. At 17 months after diagnosis his IFCC HbA$_{1c}$ had risen to 74 mmol/mol, with his insulin requirements indicating he had come out of the honeymoon period. He was undertaking four hours of ballet per day and at least four capillary blood glucose checks a day. He was given a personalised insulin correction sheet to tighten his glucose control, with insulin:carbohydrate ratios and insulin sensitivity factors adjusted for different meals and times of the day.

IFCC 74 ≡ DCCT 8.9%

NICE Guidelines: Type 1 diabetes in children and young people
HbA$_{1c}$ target: IFCC <59 mmol/mol ≡ <7.5%

12: Poor glucose control with microvascular complications

Sarah Griffiths and Parth Narendran, Senior House Officer in Diabetes (SG), Clinical Senior Lecturer and Honorary Consultant in Diabetes (PN), Birmingham, UK

Background

A 19-year-old woman, diagnosed nine years previously with type 1 diabetes was seen in the adult diabetes clinic. She had a history of poorly controlled diabetes complicated by an eating disorder, and at times would omit her insulin completely. Her IFCC HbA$_{1c}$ at this time was 148 mmol/mol.

IFCC 148 ≡ DCCT 15.7%

She had background diabetic retinopathy, markedly elevated triglyceride levels, and problems with constipation. Her most symptomatic problem at the time of review was severe shooting and burning pain in both her hands and feet, and allodynia (heightened sensitivity to touch). This pain was poorly controlled despite multiple analgesic medication, and was severe enough to keep her awake at night.

Treatment plan

The need for good glycaemic control to halt disease progression was discussed with the patient. A plan was made for insulin injections to be supervised by her grandmother.

IFCC 110 ≡ DCCT 12.2%

Two months later, her IFCC HbA$_{1c}$ had improved to 110 mmol/mol. The pain from her peripheral neuropathy persisted, however, despite additional medication, and became sufficiently troubling that three months later she was admitted to hospital for symptom control. The intensive input from the diabetic team during this period led to an improvement in blood glucose control. Repeat HbA$_{1c}$ testing one month later showed an IFCC HbA$_{1c}$ 77 mmol/mol, with more improvement two months later at 70 mmol/mol.

IFCC 77 ≡ DCCT 9.2%
IFCC 70 ≡ DCCT 8.6%

Follow-up

A year later, the pain from her diabetic neuropathy had improved and she was able to decrease her analgesic intake. Unfortunately her fears of weight gain had returned and she was again omitting insulin. She suffered from increased symptoms associated with gastroparesis and her IFCC HbA$_{1c}$ had once again risen to 132 mmol/mol.

IFCC 132 ≡ DCCT 14.2

NICE Guidelines: Type 1 diabetes in children and young people
HbA$_{1c}$ targets: IFCC 48 mmol/mol ≡ 6.5% to IFCC 59 mmol/mol ≡ 7.5%

13: Renal failure and cardiovascular disease in an Asian patient

Alex Wright, Consultant Physician, Walsall/Birmingham, UK

Background

In 1984 a 41-year-old man from India was diagnosed with type 2 diabetes. After four years of diet and lifestyle advice his diabetes was poorly controlled with an IFCC HbA$_{1c}$ 89 mmol/mol. He was hypertensive with renal impairment (serum creatinine raised at 155 µmol/l) and he had an enlarged heart. Angina was diagnosed in 1993, a myocardial infarction in 2008 and left ventricular failure in 2009 with BNP 3552 pg/ml (normal <400 pg/ml).

IFCC 89 ≡ DCCT 10.3%

His BMI, 36 kg/m^2, was unchanged from 1999 despite several attempts to reduce calorie intake and cessation of smoking. Increasing physical activity was limited by poor cardiovascular reserve. Renal function changed little over the years with normal ultrasound scans, and serum creatinine was 159 µmol/l in 2009, when metformin was discontinued. Cataracts developed but no significant retinopathy, neuropathy or peripheral vascular disease. Glycaemic control fluctuated with IFCC HbA$_{1c}$ 64 in 2000, 38 in 2003 (fructosamine 282 µmol/l), 79 in 2005, and 64 and 105 mmol/mol in 2006.

IFCC 64 ≡ DCCT 8.0%
IFCC 38 ≡ DCCT 5.6%
IFCC 79 ≡ DCCT 9.4%
IFCC 105 ≡ DCCT 11.8%

Treatment plan

From 1988 to 2006, treatment included a sulphonylurea and metformin. The sulphonylurea was discontinued in 2006 and insulin started. Blood pressure was well controlled using a calcium channel-blocking drug and beta blocker. A statin was advised in 1993 but cholesterol was still 7.8 mmol/l in 1997.

Follow-up

After insulin was started, IFCC HbA$_{1c}$ decreased to 62 and 32 mmol/mol. He was taking 25/75 mix insulin three times a day with meals with 58 units at breakfast, 24 units at midday, and 58 units in the evening. Recent haemoglobin was 9.7 g/dl with cholesterol 3.6 mmol/l.

IFCC 62 ≡ DCCT 7.8%
IFCC 32 ≡ DCCT 5.1%

If glycaemic control had been judged by HbA$_{1c}$, insulin therapy should have been started in 2005. Management would have been helped if drug compliance had been checked. Fructosamine determination was concordant with HbA$_{1c}$ in 2003, but the more recent development of anaemia associated with renal failure could have affected red cell turnover and possibly HbA$_{1c}$ values.

NICE Guidelines: Type 2 diabetes
HbA$_{1c}$ targets: IFCC 48 mmol/mol ≡ 6.5% to IFCC 59 mmol/mol ≡ 7.5%

14: Type 1 diabetes in a teenage girl concerned about weight

Julie A. Edge, Consultant in Paediatric Diabetes, Oxford, UK

Background

A previously well-controlled 14-year-old girl with type 1 diabetes had lost 3 kg in weight over three months and her IFCC HbA$_{1c}$ had climbed from 59 to 81 mmol/mol. She was on a multiple injection regimen using a preprandial rapid-acting insulin analogue with once-daily basal long-acting analogue given in the evening, and said that she was carbohydrate counting. She admitted that she had been missing most of her lunchtime insulin doses at school and occasional long-acting insulin doses.

IFCC 59 ≡ DCCT 7.5%
IFCC 81 ≡ DCCT 9.6%

Treatment plan

A different insulin regimen was selected in view of the missed doses. Because of the weight loss, gentle enquiries were made on whether she was concerned about weight and shape, and also an assessment of her mental state as depression and anxiety are more common in young people with diabetes. Her regimen was changed to a biphasic insulin in the morning, with a rapid-acting analogue at the evening meal, and long-acting analogue was continued in the evening. An outpatient appointment was made for her in a month because her HbA$_{1c}$ had risen rapidly and changes had been made.

Follow-up

Three weeks later she was admitted to hospital in severe diabetic ketoacidosis; pH 6.9, blood glucose 33.5 mmol/l and ketones 5.6 mmol/l. Her IFCC HbA$_{1c}$ had risen to 96 mmol/mol. On recovery her weight had dropped further, and she finally admitted to omitting insulin doses for the purposes of weight control. Despite psychological support and adjustments to her insulin regimen, over the next two years her IFCC HbA$_{1c}$ levels ranged from 92 to 111 mmol/mol and she had three further admissions in ketoacidosis.

IFCC 96 ≡ DCCT 10.9%

IFCC 92 ≡ DCCT 10.6%
IFCC 111 ≡ DCCT 12.3%

After the age of 17 she made some progress and her IFCC HbA$_{1c}$ level fell to 72 mmol/mol. She realised the harmful effects of high blood glucose levels, and began to feel less irritable and aggressive once she had controlled her diabetes better.

IFCC 72 ≡ DCCT 8.7%

NICE Guidelines: Type 1 diabetes in children and young people
HbA$_{1c}$ target: IFCC <59 mmol/mol ≡ <7.5%

15: Glycaemic control through patient empowerment

You Yi Hong, Máire O'Donnell and Sean F. Dinneen,
Surgical Intern (YYH), Research Associate (MO'D), Consultant Physician
(SFD), Galway, Ireland

Background

A 68-year-old man, diagnosed ten years earlier with type 2 diabetes, regularly attended the hospital diabetes clinic. He also had hypertension, dyslipidaemia and benign prostatic hyperplasia. He used pre-mixed insulin (12 units pre-breakfast and 14 units pre-tea). His medications included aspirin, atorvastatin, lansoprazole and tamsulosin. At his last clinic visit his weight was 82.8 kg and his blood pressure was 150/90 mmHg. His IFCC HbA_{1c} was

IFCC 59 ≡ DCCT 7.5%

59 mmol/mol. His lipid levels were within target and he had no evidence of complications from his diabetes. None of this information was communicated to the patient in a written format, but it was sent in writing to his GP.

Treatment plan

The patient agreed to participate in a pilot study on the impact of a one-page clinical information sheet showing personal clinical data, given to people with diabetes in the waiting room prior to their consultation. The sheet contained a brief summary of the patient's diabetes status, including recent laboratory results. A short verbal explanation of the information sheet was given, and he was encouraged to read through it before his consultation.

He was actively involved in the consultation and the clinical information sheet prompted him to raise the issue of having gained 4 kg in weight in four months. Advice and counselling regarding regular exercise was given, and he was also referred to the dietician. An ACE inhibitor was added to his list of current medication.

Follow-up

IFCC 44 ≡ DCCT 6.2%

This patient's IFCC HbA_{1c} was 44 mmol/mol three months after this review, and he was proud to have achieved a result below the IFCC HbA_{1c} target

IFCC 48 ≡ DCCT 6.5%

of 48 mmol/mol. A clinical information sheet is a good way of promoting greater patient participation during clinic visits.

NICE Guidelines: Type 2 diabetes
HbA_{1c} targets: IFCC 48 mmol/mol ≡ 6.5% to IFCC 59 mmol/mol ≡ 7.5%

16: Diagnosis and early management of type 2 diabetes in patient with acute coronary syndrome

Maggie Sinclair Hammersley and Daniel Hammersley, Consultant Physician, Oxford (MSH), Medical Student, London (DH), UK

Background

A 77-year-old man with no history of type 2 diabetes was admitted to a district general hospital with an acute ST segment elevation anterior myocardial infarction. He was found to have elevated cardiac Troponin-I >50 µg/l (reference range <1.0 µg/l); his BMI was 31 kg/m², he smoked 40 packets per year. He had an admission plasma glucose of 16 mmol/l, IFCC HbA$_{1c}$ 95 mmol/mol and cholesterol 7.3 mmol/l. He underwent thrombolysis and was started on an intravenous insulin infusion. Following persistent ST-segment elevation, he was transferred to a tertiary centre for rescue PCI (percutaneous coronary intervention, or angioplasty). An echocardiogram revealed a mildly impaired ejection fraction (45-50%), a hypokinetic anterior wall with an akinetic apex and a dilated left atrium (5.4cm).

IFCC 95 mmol/mol ≡ 10.8%

Treatment plan

He underwent successful rescue PCI with insertion of a stent to the circumflex artery. The intravenous insulin infusion was continued until 12 hours after the successful revascularisation. Insulin was then discontinued but fasting plasma glucose remained high at 10.4 mmol/l. In line with the current trust guideline following the DIGAMI study, he was started on subcutaneous insulin for three months. He was also started on once-daily treatment with clopidogrel 75 mg, aspirin 75 mg, simvastatin 40 mg, ramipril 5 mg, and bisoprolol 5 mg. He was informed of the diagnosis of diabetes, advised on lifestyle modification and discharged.

Follow-up

He was reviewed in the diabetes clinic three months later. His IFCC HbA$_{1c}$ had decreased to 75 mmol/mol. After discussion with the patient, insulin was discontinued. Two days later his fasting blood glucose was 9.9 mmol/l and his home blood glucose monitoring showed 8.5–15.8 mmol/l. He was started on metformin, in increments up to 1 g twice daily. Over the following three months, gliclazide was added at 80 mg once daily to attain the target for IFCC HbA$_{1c}$ recommended by NICE of <59 mmol/mol.

IFCC 75 mmol/mol ≡ 9.0%

IFCC 59 mmol/mol ≡ 7.5%

NICE Guidelines: Type 2 diabetes
HbA$_{1c}$ targets: IFCC 48 mmol/mol ≡ 6.5% to IFCC 59 mmol/mol ≡ 7.5%

17: Incretin or insulin?

Richard Paisey, Consultant Physician, Torbay, UK

Background

A 43-year-old lorry driver was diagnosed with type 2 diabetes during a routine health check. At that time he weighed 86 kg, BMI was 33 kg/m², and blood pressure was 140/85 mmHg. Blood tests revealed fasting blood glucose 8.3 mmol/l, cholesterol 5.2 mmol/l and triglycerides 2.9 mmol/l, creatinine 82 µmol/l and IFCC HbA$_{1c}$ 78 mmol/mol. Five years later, the recent addition of gliclazide to metformin had resulted in a fall in IFCC HbA$_{1c}$ to 69 mmol/mol, but also a 4 kg weight gain. There was a good response to simvastatin: cholesterol was 3.9 mmol/l. Ramipril 10 mg daily achieved blood pressure of 130/65 mmHg.

IFCC 78 ≡ DCCT 9.3%
IFCC 69 ≡ DCCT 8.5%

Treatment plan

His HGV driving licence, which was already in jeopardy because of the risk of hypoglycaemia with sulphonylurea, would have been revoked if insulin had been introduced. Incretin therapy was discussed, and the patient agreed to try subcutaneous exenatide 5 µg twice daily for one month and, if tolerated, to increase the dose to 10 µg twice daily.

Follow-up

Gliclazide was discontinued after one month as blood glucose levels were all 5–10 mmol/l. Exenatide was increased to 10 µg twice daily, with advice to discontinue in the case of nausea and vomiting, and to seek immediate advice if abdominal pains occurred because of the possible rare association with pancreatitis. After six months on metformin and exenatide he felt well, with only occasional nausea after a main meal. He had lost 5 kg in weight and his IFCC HbA$_{1c}$ had decreased to 41 mmol/mol without any evidence of hypoglycaemia on home blood glucose monitoring or symptoms.

IFCC 41 ≡ DCCT 5.9%

He had informed the DVLA of the treatment change and was granted his HGV licence, with advice to submit to a full diabetes review in one year. He was encouraged to keep his imminent retinal screening appointment, in view of the relatively rapid improvement in glycaemic control. His GP was asked to take over exenatide prescription under the local shared care plan.

NICE Guidelines: Type 2 diabetes
HbA$_{1c}$ targets: IFCC 48 mmol/mol ≡ 6.5% to IFCC 59 mmol/mol ≡ 7.5%

18: Type 2 diabetes and pregnancy

Nick Lewis-Barned, Consultant Physician and Senior Lecturer,
Northumbria, UK

Background

A 34-year-old Chinese woman, BMI 32 kg/m² had been diagnosed with type
2 diabetes three years previously. She started on metformin treatment after
two and a half years because her IFCC HbA$_{1c}$ was 66 mmol/mol. Since then
her periods became more regular and she unexpectedly found that she was
nine weeks pregnant. Her GP measured her HbA$_{1c}$ (IFCC 54 mmol/mol) and
referred her to the joint antenatal diabetes clinic.

IFCC 66 ≡ DCCT 8.1%

IFCC 54 ≡ DCCT 7.1%

Treatment plan

She was started on folic acid treatment (5 mg daily) and introduced to the
specialist team. In consultation with a specialist dietician she identified
a number of food-related changes that she could make. She also met the
specialist midwife and learned how to start self-monitoring of her blood
glucose.

Follow-up

She was reviewed after two weeks and her self-monitored glucose levels were
all within target range (fasting below 5 mmol/l and postprandial below
7.5 mmol/l). A further two weeks later her IFCC HbA$_{1c}$ was 40 mmol/mol.

IFCC 40 ≡ DCCT 5.9%

At about 18 weeks' gestation her glucose levels had drifted higher than the
target range and her IFCC HbA$_{1c}$ had risen to 52 mmol/mol. A decision was
taken to transfer her to prandial insulin and to stop her metformin. Her
HbA$_{1c}$ returned to IFCC 36 mmol/mol, and her glucose levels remained well
controlled without hypoglycaemia through the rest of her pregnancy.

IFCC 52 ≡ DCCT 6.9%

IFCC 36 ≡ DCCT 5.5%

Following delivery, insulin was discontinued. While she was able to keep
to her dietary changes, her HbA$_{1c}$ remained at 46 mmol/mol. However, she
found this difficult to maintain , and after three months her HbA$_{1c}$ had risen
to 58 mmol/mol and metformin was restarted.

IFCC 46 ≡ DCCT 6.4%

IFCC 58 ≡ DCCT 7.5%

NICE Guidelines: Diabetes in pregnancy
HbA$_{1c}$ target prepregnancy*: IFCC <43 mmol/mol ≡ <6.1%
*(if safely achievable)

19: Deterioration of pre-existing diabetes in a patient on low dose quetiapine

Valeria Frighi and Matthew Stephenson, Senior Clinical Researcher (VF), Consultant Psychiatrist in Learning Disability (MS), Oxford, UK

Background

A 39-year-old insulin-treated man with type 2 diabetes, learning disability and schizophrenia treated with haloperidol 4 mg, was started on quetiapine (100 mg daily). His glycaemic control had been excellent since soon after the diabetes diagnosis four years previously, with IFCC HbA$_{1c}$ between 34 and 40 mmol/mol, and home blood glucose levels of 5–7 mmol/l on long-acting insulin 10 units daily.

IFCC 34 ≡ DCCT 5.3%
IFCC 40 ≡ DCCT 5.8%

Within two weeks of initiation of quetiapine, the patient developed hyperglycaemic symptoms, with glucoses of 10–20 mmol/l. His GP referred him to the diabetic clinic, where IFCC HbA$_{1c}$ was recorded as 87 mmol/mol with the patient on 30 units of insulin daily. The patient's weight was stable, with a BMI of 32 kg/m^2.

IFCC 87 ≡ DCCT 10.1%

Treatment and follow-up

The GP was advised to increase the insulin dose gradually. Six months later, the patient, on 38 units of insulin daily, was seen again in the diabetic clinic with IFCC HbA1 of 81 mmol/mol. At this stage, quetiapine was stopped. Glucose levels were not initially reduced after quetiapine withdrawal, despite an increase in insulin up to 50 units daily. However, 23 days after quetiapine withdrawal and ten days after the introduction of metformin, blood glucose started to fall very rapidly. Insulin was quickly down-titrated to 16 units daily. IFCC HbA$_{1c}$ fell, to 50 mmol/mol after one month and 53 mmol/mol after two months. Within three months, metabolic control had returned to the levels seen before the introduction of quetiapine, and the patient was fit to undergo general surgery. Glycaemic control remained excellent two years later with IFCC HbA$_{1c}$ around 40 mmol/mol, and the patient on metformin 850 mg twice daily. He was maintained on haloperidol monotherapy throughout, with no deterioration in his mental state at any stage.

IFCC 81 ≡ DCCT 9.6%

IFCC 50 ≡ DCCT 6.7%
IFCC 53 ≡ DCCT 7.0%

IFCC 40 ≡ DCCT 5.8%

This case confirms current evidence that atypical antipsychotics can exacerbate pre-existing diabetes or induce it *de novo*. It also shows the usefulness of HbA$_{1c}$ for appropriate clinical management.

NICE Guidelines: Type 2 diabetes
HbA$_{1c}$ targets: IFCC 48 mmol/mol ≡ 6.5% to IFCC 59 mmol/mol ≡ 7.5%

20: Low HbA$_{1c}$ and risk of hypoglycaemia

Jonathan Roland, Consultant Diabetologist, Peterborough, UK

Background

A 50-year-old woman was referred because of frequent debilitating hypoglycaemia and loss of hypoglycaemic warning signs. She had been diagnosed
with type 1 diabetes at the age of two, but had only recently moved to the
locality. She had severe retinopathy, for which she had received extensive
laser treatment; leaving her with vision of 6/6 in the right eye and counting
fingers in her left. Despite the long duration of diabetes she did not have
microalbuminuria and was not troubled by neuropathy. Her IFCC HbA$_{1c}$
was 35 mmol/mol. She felt her previous medical advisers had blamed her for   IFCC 35 ≡ DCCT 5.4%
keeping her diabetes poorly controlled and this was the reason she had lost
her vision in her right eye. She felt very guilty whenever her blood glucose
went above 7 mmol/l, and was terrified of losing the sight in her remaining
eye.

Treatment

The risks of hypoglycaemia were explained to her; as were the limited
benefits that meticulous control was likely to bring her, given the length of
time she had already had diabetes. She was offered a structured education
program for insulin dose adjustment according to carbohydrate intake, and
was advised to keep her blood glucose always above 4 mmol/l. Frequent oph-
thalmological screening was organised to avoid problems in her remaining
eye.

Follow-up

Initially she kept herself hypoglycaemic, but was eventually able to gain the
confidence to start relaxing her control and regard a blood glucose level of
7 mmol/l as an acceptable average rather than a maximum. Her IFCC HbA$_{1c}$
now runs between 43 and 51 mmol/mol. Her hypoglycaemia has become   IFCC 43 ≡ DCCT 6.1%
much less frequent and because some warning signs have now returned, this   IFCC 51 ≡ DCCT 6.8%
is much less of a problem to her.

NICE Guidelines: Type 1 diabetes in adults
HbA$_{1c}$ targets: IFCC 48 mmol/mol ≡ 6.5% to IFCC 59 mmol/mol ≡ 7.5%

21: Rapid changes in glycaemic control and retinopathy

Adele Farnsworth and Alex Wright, Lead Diabetic Retinal Screener (AF),
Consultant Physician (AW), Walsall/Birmingham, UK

Background

IFCC 68 ≡ DCCT 8.4%
IFCC 97 ≡ DCCT 11.0%

A 23-year-old woman presented to the antenatal clinic with an unplanned pregnancy at 12 weeks' gestation. Type 1 diabetes had been diagnosed at the age of 10 years, and had been managed on twice daily 30/70 mix insulin. Attendance in the paediatric, transitional and young persons' diabetes clinics was sporadic and glycated haemoglobin showed suboptimal glycaemic control. IFCC HbA$_{1c}$ ranged between 68 mmol/mol at best, to a more usual level of 97 mmol/mol. During this time, three episodes of diabetic ketoacidosis occurred without any clear precipitating factors, and her compliance with monitoring and her insulin regimen was questioned. Basal bolus insulin was tried for a few weeks, but after another episode of ketoacidosis, treatment was changed back to twice daily 30/70 mix.

Treatment plan

IFCC 91 ≡ DCCT 10.5%

IFCC 86 ≡ DCCT 10.0%
IFCC 77 ≡ DCCT 9.2%
IFCC 74 ≡ DCCT 8.9%
IFCC 68 ≡ DCCT 8.4%
IFCC 63 ≡ DCCT 7.9%
IFCC 57 ≡ DCCT 7.4%

At antenatal booking, IFCC HbA$_{1c}$ was 91 mmol/mol. Her partner was supportive and was encouraged to become involved in her diabetes management, with a change back to basal bolus insulin and carbohydrate counting. At subsequent fortnightly visits IFCC HbA$_{1c}$ was 86, 77, 74, 68, 63 and 57 mmol/mol.

Follow-up

At 24 weeks' gestation some blurring of vision was reported and repeat retinal photography showed R3/M1 grade proliferative retinopathy/maculopathy with peripheral new vessels. Worsening of retinopathy may result from large and rapid changes in glycaemic control. Retinal photography is suggested when a fall in DCCT HbA$_{1c}$ of 3% or more is anticipated; this would equate to a fall of approximately 30 mmol/mol in IFCC units.

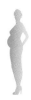

NICE Guidelines: Diabetes in pregnancy
HbA$_{1c}$ target prepregnancy*: IFCC <43 mmol/mol ≡ <6.1%
*(if safely achievable)

22: Type 1 diabetes in a young man moving from paediatric to young adult services

Nick Lewis-Barned, Consultant Physician and Senior Lecturer,
Northumbria, UK

Background

A 15-year-old young man, who had developed type 1 diabetes at the age of eight, had become increasingly withdrawn in consultations. This had become more pronounced over the previous two years. His mother was worried that he was not looking after his diabetes properly and was staying out late with his friends. Despite being on a regime of four daily insulin injections (evening long acting and short acting before meals) his HbA_{1c} over a nine-month period was IFCC HbA_{1c} 70, 86 and finally 92 mmol/mol.

IFCC 70 ≡ DCCT 8.6%
IFCC 86 ≡ DCCT 10.0%
IFCC 92 ≡ DCCT 10.6%

Treatment plan

As part of transitional care, he met with a member of the team on his own, to discuss changes he wanted to make in preparation for moving into the young adult service, and what support he needed from the clinical teams. He said he was embarrassed at giving insulin at school, and missed midday doses. He also wanted to be able to go out with his friends or play sport in the evenings, and felt his parents were always 'on his case'. He was worried about having hypos while he was with his friends. He decided to try a premixed insulin in the morning on school days and asked if he could be seen on his own in the clinic sometimes. He had a lot of questions about his diabetes, which he did not like to admit in front of his parents.

Follow-up

Over the next nine months, he met with team members on two occasions and also had some telephone follow-up. His confidence in dealing with his diabetes grew; he felt able to let a few of his close friends know about it and actively varied his insulin amounts around food and physical activity. His blood glucose fell with IFCC HbA_{1c} 62 mmol/mol, and he was pleased with the improvement. He decided not to make any more changes at the present time.

IFCC 62mmol/mol ≡ DCCT 7.8%

NICE Guidelines: Type 1 diabetes in children and young people
HbA_{1c} target: IFCC <59 mmol/mol ≡ <7.5%

23: Monitoring glycaemic control: HbA_{1c} or fructosamine

Sarah Moore, GP, Worcestershire, UK

Background

A 72-year-old Caucasian man diagnosed with type 2 diabetes in 1999 was under follow-up care in general practice. Review of his glycaemic control since 2004 revealed that he had persistent glycosuria, raised blood glucose ranging from 22.7 to 24.9 mmol/l, but with an IFCC HbA_{1c} level of between 44 and 46 mmol/mol.

IFCC 44 ≡ DCCT 6.2%
IFCC 46 ≡ DCCT 6.4%

He had a history of polycythaemia rubra vera which had been treated with ^{32}P since 1978, but was not currently needing any treatment. He also suffered from thrombocytopenia and peripheral vascular disease with a right femoral tibial arterial bypass, renal calculus, recurrent DVT, chronic interstitial cystitis, chronic urticaria, acne rosacea and alcohol excess. He was not on any treatment; refusing to be on long-term warfarin as it aggravated the chronic interstitial cystitis.

Treatment plan

In 2007, as he had persistently raised blood sugar but with HbA_{1c} in normal range, his case was discussed with the clinical biochemist as to whether it was appropriate to be monitoring his glycaemic control with HbA_{1c} in view of his past history of polycythaemia rubra vera. Further tests showed a raised fructosamine level (400 μmol/l), normal haemoglobin, a raised reticulocyte count (139.8×10^9/l) and a blood film which showed polychromatic cells and a few spherocytes. He was started on metformin, but did not tolerate this and is now controlled on gliclazide 80 mg.

Follow-up

As the patient has accelerated turnover of red blood cells due to polycythaemia rubra vera, the HbA_{1c} test does not accurately reflect glycaemic control. His blood glucose is now monitored using fructosamine. Contra-indications for using HbA_{1c} include polycythaemias, other anaemias, presence of haemoglobin variants, pregnancy, venesection or recent blood transfusion.

NICE Guidelines: Type 2 diabetes
HbA_{1c} targets: IFCC 48 mmol/mol ≡ 6.5% to IFCC 59 mmol/mol ≡ 7.5%

24: Prepregnancy and pregnancy in type 1 diabetes

Ciara McLaughlin and David R. McCance, Specialist Registrar (CM),
Honorary Professor of Endocrinology/Consultant Physician (DRM),
Belfast, Northern Ireland, UK

Background

A 28-year-old woman with a 16-year history of type 1 diabetes, attending her routine diabetes clinic appointment, expressed a wish to become pregnant. She was using the oral contraceptive pill and smoked 20 cigarettes per day. Her IFCC HbA_{1c} was 66 mmol/mol and she performed only occasional home glucose monitoring. Her diabetes was controlled on a basal bolus regimen of insulin aspart and detemir. She had documented background retinopathy and was taking an ACE inhibitor for microalbuminuria.

IFCC 66 ≡ DCCT 8.2%

Treatment plan

Prepregnancy planning was undertaken with particular reference to her poor diabetic control, cigarette smoking and microvascular complications, and to take into account that her treatment with an ACE inhibitor was contraindicated in pregnancy. The priority was for her to remain on contraception until her diabetic control improved: the NICE guidelines recommend an IFCC HbA_{1c} of <43 mmol/mol, if safe, preconception.

IFCC 43 ≡ DCCT 6.1%

She was offered advice on diet, lifestyle and smoking cessation, started on folic acid 5 mg daily, reminded of the need for daily capillary glucose monitoring (and the targets) and referred to an ophthalmologist. Methyldopa was substituted for her ACE inhibitor.

Follow-up

Following implementation of these measures, regular clinic visits and telephone contact with the diabetic nurse specialist for insulin adjustment, her IFCC HbA_{1c} fell over the following three months to 53 mmol/mol, with capillary glucose results on target. She subsequently discontinued her contraception. At conception four months later, her IFCC HbA_{1c} was 51 mmol/mol and she was referred urgently to the joint diabetes antenatal clinic for ongoing care. Her IFCC HbA_{1c} at the end of the first trimester was 48 mmol/mol and remained between 37 and 42 mmol/mol for the remainder of the pregnancy. She gave birth to a health baby boy weighing 3.9 kg by elective caesarean section at 38 weeks gestation.

IFCC 53 ≡ DCCT 7.0%

IFCC 51 ≡ DCCT 6.8%

IFCC 48 ≡ DCCT 6.5%
IFCC 37 ≡ DCCT 5.5%
IFCC 42 ≡ DCCT 6.0%

> NICE Guidelines: Diabetes in pregnancy
> **HbA_{1c} target prepregnancy*: IFCC <43 mmol/mol ≡ <6.1%**
> *(if safely achievable)

25: Maturity onset diabetes of the young, subtype *HNF1A* (*HNF1A*-MODY)

Amanda Webster and Katharine R. Owen, Genetic Diabetes Specialist Nurse (AW), Clinician Scientist (KRO), Oxford, UK

Background

A young woman aged 21 was diagnosed opportunistically with type 1 diabetes in 2001, and basal-bolus insulin was started. Her mother had been diagnosed with type 2 diabetes during pregnancy when aged 24 years, and was currently being treated with oral hypoglycaemic agents.

IFCC 60 ≡ DCCT 7.6%
IFCC 77 ≡ DCCT 9.2%

Subsequently, the young woman's attendance at clinic was sporadic. Her insulin dose increased to 0.8 units/kg, with IFCC HbA$_{1c}$ ranging from 60 to 77 mmol/mol over the following six years. She was depressed about her erratic control, and her weight increased by 18 kg to 80 kg (BMI 30.1 kg/m^2).

In 2007, her brother was diagnosed with type 2 diabetes, aged 25 years. The striking family history led to the aetiology of the young woman's diabetes being questioned. Investigations revealed a normal random C-peptide level at 0.49 nmol/l (fasting reference range 0.27–1.28 nmol/l), indicating endogenous insulin secretion; hence type 1 diabetes was unlikely. Molecular genetic testing was arranged, revealing a mutation in *HNF1A*, causing maturity onset diabetes of the young (MODY) in all the family members diagnosed with diabetes.

Treatment plan

IFCC 40 ≡ DCCT 5.8%

The treatment of choice for *HNF1A*-MODY is low-dose sulphonylurea drugs. This patient's basal-bolus insulin was discontinued and gliclazide 40 mg once daily started. Stopping insulin caused great anxiety to the patient, so she received daily contact from the diabetic specialist nurse and 24-hour phone support was available through the on-call clinical team. The treatment change progressed without problems and IFCC HbA$_{1c}$ was 40 mmol/mol after five months, with no hypoglycaemia reported.

Follow-up

IFCC 38 ≡ DCCT 5.6%
IFCC 42 ≡ DCCT 6.0%

Two years later IFCC HbA$_{1c}$ was stable at 38–42 mmol/mol on gliclazide 40 mg once daily. She lost the weight (18 kg) she had gained while on insulin. She was followed up regularly in the monogenic diabetes clinic with no evidence of any diabetic complications.

NICE Guidelines: Type 2 diabetes
HbA$_{1c}$ targets: IFCC 48 mmol/mol ≡ 6.5% to IFCC 59 mmol/mol ≡ 7.5%

26: 'Overtreating' type 2 diabetes

Simon Heller, Professor of Clinical Diabetes, Sheffield, UK

Background

A 69-year-old lady, living alone with early dementia, had been diagnosed with type 2 diabetes two years earlier following a routine glucose tolerance test. She had a BMI of 25 kg/m², a 10-year history of hypertension and had recovered well from a mild stroke five years earlier. She had no microvascular complications. She had been started on metformin (1 g twice daily) and her IFCC HbA$_{1c}$ of 62 mmol/mol fell to between 48 and 53 mmol/mol. Her serum creatinine had gradually risen from 110 to 160 μmol/l, probably due to her hypertensive renal disease. Her GP had recently stopped her metformin and started 80 mg gliclazide twice daily.

IFCC 62 ≡ DCCT 7.8%
IFCC 48 ≡ DCCT 6.5%
IFCC 53 ≡ DCCT 7.0%

Four weeks later, her daughter contacted the practice urgently, stating that for the last week her mother had been more confused and forgetful than usual. She regularly measured her mother's blood glucose using a meter she had bought herself (the practice only supported blood testing for patients on insulin as it was of 'no value' in other patients with type 2 diabetes). On three out of four occasions throughout one day it had been between 2 and 3 mmol/l.

Treatment plan

The practice nurse told the daughter to stop the gliclazide therapy immediately and arranged to see the patient on the following day. She found her to be extremely confused, although a random blood glucose measurement was 7 mmol/l. She took blood which subsequently returned an IFCC HbA$_{1c}$ result of 41 mmol/mol.

IFCC 41 ≡ DCCT 5.9%

Follow-up

Over the following days the patient's confusion largely resolved, although her short-term memory remained poor. She had no symptoms of poorly controlled diabetes. Fasting glucose, measured at home by her daughter stayed between 7 and 9 mmol/l. Two determinations in the following six months showed IFCC HbA$_{1c}$ 60–62 mmol/mol. It was agreed that she should remain on dietary treatment alone.

IFCC 60 ≡ DCCT 7.6%
IFCC 62 ≡ DCCT 7.8%

NICE Guidelines: Type 2 diabetes
HbA$_{1c}$ targets: IFCC 48 mmol/mol ≡ 6.5% to IFCC 59 mmol/mol ≡ 7.5%

27: Diabetes and an elevated triglyceride concentration

Robert Cramb, Consultant Chemical Pathologist, Birmingham, UK

Background

A 48-year-old man was referred to the lipid clinic. He had been diagnosed with diabetes eight months previously, but had no other significant past medical history. He had no evidence of heart disease and his weight had been decreasing. His mother had diabetes for ten years and developed angina in the five years prior to her death, aged 69 years. Despite taking metformin in a slow release preparation, the patient's IFCC HbA$_{1C}$ was 99 mmol/mol. His serum cholesterol was elevated at 7.0 mmol/l and also his triglyceride concentration at 6.8 mmol/l.

IFCC 99 ≡ DCCT 11.2%

Treatment plan

A low dose of fenofibrate was prescribed at 67 mg once daily, which caused a drop in both his cholesterol concentration to 5.6 mmol/l and triglycerides to 2.6 mmol/l. Since his mother had developed angina before the age of 65 years, he was considered to be at risk of cardiovascular disease. For this reason, he was prescribed a statin, rosuvastatin in a low dose (10 mg), as well as a fibrate to decrease his cholesterol concentration further.

Follow-up

By the time he was seen in the lipid clinic four months later, he was also taking gliclazide at a dosage of 80 mg once daily, to improve the control of his diabetes. His cholesterol was 3.6 mmol/l and his triglyceride concentration 2.1 mmol/l. His IFCC HbA$_{1C}$ had been reduced to 63 mmol/mol.

IFCC 63 ≡ DCCT 7.9%

Treatment with a combination of fibrate and statin can cause myositis but rarely leads to rhabdomyolysis. However, in patients with diabetes and inadequately controlled mixed dyslipidaemia, despite statin therapy, the addition of a fibrate can markedly improve lipid and glycaemic control. Patients should discontinue therapy and report for review if they develop muscle aches.

NICE Guidelines: Type 2 diabetes
HbA$_{1c}$ targets: IFCC 48 mmol/mol ≡ 6.5% to IFCC 59 mmol/mol ≡ 7.5%

28: Multiple therapies leading to bariatric surgery

Ernesto Lopez and R. David Leslie, Medical Student (EL), Professor of
Diabetes and Autoimmunity (RDL), London, UK

Background

A Caucasian man was diagnosed with diabetes in 1995 aged 24, at which
time he had no family history, no weight loss, no ketonuria and high blood
glucose. At that time he was obese (BMI $37.2\,kg/m^2$ and weighed $109.8\,kg$),
his blood pressure was $147/73\,mmHg$ and IFCC HbA_{1c} $55\,mmol/mol$. To
define the nature of his diabetes he was checked for diabetes-associated
autoantibodies (all negative), MODY genes (not present) and haemoglobinopathy (none detected). He presented in 2009 with an HbA_{1c} out of control
despite treatment (IFCC HbA_{1c} 98 while his personal target was $<53\,mmol/$
mol). He gave a history of psoriasis, hypertension which is well controlled
with lisinopril/indapamide, hypercholesterolemia treated with simvastatin
and a psychiatric illness treated with risperidone/citalopram.

IFCC 55 ≡ DCCT 7.1%

IFCC 98 ≡ DCCT 11.1%
IFCC 53 ≡ DCCT 7.0%

Treatment plan

After diagnosis, he had been treated with insulin (IFCC HbA_{1c} $82\,mmol/$
mol) and, subsequently, in 1999 with a multiple insulin regime plus metformin (IFCC HbA_{1c} $40\,mmol/mol$). Despite escalating insulin doses and the
introduction of a long-acting insulin analogue, his IFCC HbA_{1c} became and
remained high ($96\,mmol/mol$). In 2006 rosiglitazone was added to insulin
without success (IFCC HbA_{1c} $105\,mmol/mol$). Rosiglitazone was stopped in
2008 (IFCC HbA_{1c} $116\,mmol/mol$) and exenatide was started (out of license)
with his insulin. By 2009 persistent nausea, as an exenatide side effect, was
not resolved and exenatide was stopped; his IFCC HbA_{1c} was $98\,mmol/mol$.

IFCC 82 ≡ DCCT 9.7%

IFCC 40 ≡ DCCT 5.8%

IFCC 96 ≡ DCCT 10.9%
IFCC 105 ≡ DCCT 11.8%
IFCC 116 ≡ DCCT 12.8%

IFCC 98 ≡ DCCT 11.1%

Follow-up

Despite the different forms of therapy, he remained generally unwell, depressed, tired, and with IFCC HbA_{1c} values for years after diagnosis between
82 and $116\,mmol/mol$. His BMI increased from 37 to $41\,kg/m^2$, with his
weight at $121.4\,kg$. His total cholesterol remained high ($4.6\,mmol/l$) while
his aim was $4.0\,mmol/l$; despite simvastatin $40\,mg$. He was referred for
evaluation for bariatric surgery.

IFCC 82 ≡ DCCT 9.7%
IFCC 116 ≡ DCCT 12.8%

NICE Guidelines: Type 2 diabetes
HbA$_{1c}$ targets: IFCC 48 mmol/mol ≡ 6.5% to IFCC 59 mmol/mol ≡ 7.5%

Richard Paisey and Rob Willox, Consultant Physician (RP), Retinal Screening Technician (RW), Torbay, UK

Background

IFCC 88 ≡ DCCT 10.2%

A 19-year-old man had been diagnosed with type 1 diabetes aged five, when he presented with ketoacidosis. His IFCC HbA$_{1c}$ was 88 mmol/mol and BMI 29 kg/m^2, blood pressure 140/90 mmHg and his urine tested positive for microalbuminuria. Retinal screening identified microaneurysms which were under three-monthly review and his VA (visual acuity) remained at 6/6 for each eye. He was referred urgently to the ophthalmology clinic because of sudden reduced VA in his left eye. This had fallen to 6/36 with the optic disc swollen, and some progression of macular changes but no oedema. The eye was highly hypermetropic with a very crowded disc (see Plate 1, page 75). An MRI brain scan excluded demyelination. Blood tests revealed serum cholesterol 5.9 mmol/l, HDL cholesterol 1.2 mmol/l, triglycerides 2.5 mmol/l, IFCC

IFCC 92 ≡ DCCT 10.6%

HbA$_{1c}$ 92 mmol/mol. Renal, hepatic and thyroid function tests were normal.

Treatment plan

Rapid improvement in glycaemic control was felt inadvisable because the potential reduction in retinal blood flow could worsen the retinal problems. He was therefore encouraged to improve his diet, while maintaining the four-times-daily insulin regimen. He was started on an ACE inhibitor and simvastatin. VA stabilised at 6/36 in the left eye and 6/6 in the right. Two weeks later bezafibrate was introduced for treatment of mild hyperlipidaemia.

Follow-up

Two months later VA in his eye had improved to 6/18 and the optic disc swelling had lessened. Blood pressure was 120/70 mmHg; IFCC HbA$_{1c}$

IFCC 78 ≡ DCCT 9.6%

78 mmol/mol, serum cholesterol 3.4 mmol/l, HDL cholesterol 1.3 mmol/l, triglycerides 1.1 mmol/l. During the following year, retinal photocoagulation was required and visual acuity remained stable. Blood glucose levels remained at 7–11 mmol/l without serious hypoglycaemia; IFCC HbA$_{1c}$ was

IFCC 68 ≡ DCCT 8.4%

68 mmol/mol. His susceptibility to microvascular complications made it likely that he would require renal or renal/pancreas transplantation in early mid-life. Emphasis on safe, moderately good glycaemic control (IFCC HbA$_{1c}$

IFCC 60 ≡ DCCT 7.6%

60–68 mmol/mol) was appropriate. Tight control of serum lipids and blood pressure would slow renal impairment and reduce atherosclerosis.

NICE Guidelines: Type 1 diabetes in children and young people
HbA$_{1c}$ targets: IFCC 48 mmol/mol ≡ 6.5%, IFCC 59 mmol/mol ≡ 7.5%

30: Uncertainty around the estimate of average plasma glucose from HbA$_{1c}$

Eric S. Kilpatrick, Honorary Professor in Clinical Biochemistry, Hull, UK

Background

A 66-year-old woman, diagnosed with type 2 diabetes for 11 years, had no retinopathy on retinal photos and normal urinary albumin measurements. Her glycaemia was initially controlled by diet alone, but had required increasing doses of oral agents. Despite being on maximal doses of metformin, sulphonylurea and thiazolidenedione, her IFCC HbA$_{1c}$ was suboptimal at 68 mmol/mol. The decision was taken to start a single injection of isophane insulin, while at the same time discontinuing the sulphonylurea and thiazolidenedione. Six months later, after titration of her insulin dose based largely on a three-month IFCC HbA$_{1c}$ of 60 mmol/mol, the HbA$_{1c}$ had improved to 53 mmol/mol. However, the patient suffered from repeated hypoglycaemic episodes (two to three per week), which were variable in severity and at no consistent time of day. Her home blood glucose monitoring showed premeal glucose values varied between 4 and 6 mmol/l with the occasional postprandial measurement being no higher than 8 mmol/l.

FCC 68 ≡ DCCT 8.4%

IFCC 60 ≡ DCCT 7.6%
IFCC 53 ≡ DCCT 7.0%

Treatment plan

The patient's GP was aware that although the mean glucose (eAG) for a patient with an IFCC HbA$_{1c}$ value of 53 mmol/mol was around 8.6 mmol/l, it can vary between individuals from 6.8 to 10.3 mmol/l. The GP decided that this woman was likely to be closer to the lower end of this range so reduced her insulin dose by 10%, recognising that it might lead to a deterioration in glycaemic control. It was also recommended that the patient should measure her postprandial glucose more often to see if she was particularly hyperglycaemic at these times.

IFCC 53 ≡ DCCT 7.0%

Follow-up

On review three months later the patient's hypoglycaemic episodes had stopped immediately after the insulin dose reduction. Her IFCC HbA$_{1c}$ had risen to 58 mmol/mol and her premeal blood glucose values by about 1 mmol/l. Her postprandial glucose values again seldom exceeded 8 mmol/l. The decision was made to leave her treatment unchanged, accepting that the HbA$_{1c}$ value, although above the target set in the NICE guidelines, was probably appropriate in this case.

IFCC 58 ≡ DCCT 7.5%

NICE Guidelines: Type 2 diabetes
HbA$_{1c}$ targets: IFCC 48 mmol/mol ≡ 6.5% to IFCC 59 mmol/mol ≡ 7.5%

31: Antipsychotics

Richard I. G. Holt, Professor in Diabetes and Endocrinology, Southampton, UK

Background

A 35-year-old man with a history of stable chronic schizophrenia presented with excessive thirst and frequent urination. He had a family history of diabetes, was unemployed, and tended to eat a diet high in fat and refined carbohydrate. He was overweight, with a BMI of 33.9 kg/m². He had been receiving treatment with risperidone, an atypical antipsychotic, for eight years.

IFCC 100 ≡ DCCT 11.3% Type 2 diabetes was diagnosed on the basis of a random glucose determination of 13.4 mmol/l. His initial IFCC HbA$_{1c}$ was 100 mmol/mol.

Treatment plan

He was initially treated with lifestyle advice in a group setting at the community mental health trust. He succeeded in losing 8 kg in weight over three months (reaching BMI 31.4 kg/m²) and his repeat IFCC HbA$_{1c}$ fell

IFCC 72 ≡ DCCT 8.7% to 72 mmol/mol. At this point he began treatment with metformin which he tolerated well, and his IFCC HbA$_{1c}$ after a further three months was

IFCC 58 ≡ DCCT 7.5% 58 mmol/mol.

He remained well for the next six months and then suffered a relapse in his psychotic state. He was no longer able to pay attention to his diabetes management and frequently forgot his metformin. His antipsychotic medication was switched to olanzapine and his condition stabilised. An IFCC HbA$_{1c}$ test

IFCC 84 ≡ DCCT 9.8% shortly after his relapse showed it had risen to 84 mmol/mol.

Once mentally well, he was able to start taking his metformin again and

IFCC 64 ≡ DCCT 8.0% three months later his IFCC HbA$_{1c}$ had fallen again to 64 mmol/mol, despite a 3 kg weight gain.

Follow-up

Efforts were made to help him further with lifestyle modification, and sitagliptin 100 mg was added. He succeeded in bringing his IFCC HbA$_{1c}$ back

IFCC 55 ≡ DCCT 7.2% down to 55 mmol/mol.

NICE Guidelines: Type 2 diabetes
HbA$_{1c}$ targets: IFCC 48 mmol/mol ≡ 6.5% to IFCC 59 mmol/mol ≡ 7.5%

32: Abnormal liver function in a patient with type 2 diabetes

Joanne Morling, Specialty Registrar in Public Health, Edinburgh, Scotland, UK

Background

A 64-year-old man with type 2 diabetes was seen for annual review in the diabetes clinic, five years after diagnosis. Since then his diabetes had been managed with diet and metformin 500 mg three times daily. His diabetes control had been variable and a recent IFCC HbA_{1c} was 66 mmol/mol. He had been receiving simvastatin 40 mg lipid-lowering therapy for four years, and when seen his cholesterol was 3.6 mmol/l. His alcohol consumption was about 15 units per week. He was obese, with BMI 36 kg/m^2.

IFCC 66 ≡ DCCT 8.2%

Liver enzymes showed ALT 186 IU/l, ALP 98 IU/l (reference ranges ALT 10–50 IU/l and ALP 40–125 IU/l), bilirubin 21 µmol/l, albumin 42 g/l and total protein 84 g/l. Urea, creatinine, and electrolytes were within the laboratory reference ranges. Two years earlier, ALT had been 88 IU/l.

Treatment plan

Non-alcoholic fatty liver disease is common amongst people with type 2 diabetes; however this is a diagnosis of exclusion and should not be immediately assumed. A detailed history was taken confirming no recent travel or tattoos. The patient underwent repeat liver function testing six weeks later, with no change in the results. An abdominal ultrasound scan showed moderate fatty liver disease. A liver screen returned negative results for autoantibody screen (including antimitochondrial and antinuclear antibodies) and for hepatitis viral serology; alpha 1-antitrypsin was 1.2 g/l and ferritin 1080 mg/l (reference ranges A1AT 0.8–2.0 g/l and ferritin 20–250 mg/l).

Follow-up

The patient was encouraged to lose weight through a healthy diet and increased physical activity. He was counselled about the association of diabetes, obesity and fatty liver disease. It was felt unlikely that his statin therapy was responsible for his liver function derangement, and it was continued. Non-alcoholic fatty liver disease was diagnosed and it is planned for this patient to undergo annual liver function test review. There are no plans at this time for referral to hepatology or for liver biopsy, however, should his liver function deteriorate further, this would be the next step.

NICE Guidelines: Type 2 diabetes
HbA_{1c} targets: IFCC 48 mmol/mol ≡ 6.5% to IFCC 59 mmol/mol ≡ 7.5%

33: Fructosamine in diabetic nephropathy

Stuart A. Ritchie, John A. McKnight and Susan E. Manley,
Specialist Registrar (SAR), Consultant Physician (JAM), Edinburgh,
Scotland, Clinical Scientist (SEM), Birmingham, UK

Background

A 66-year-old South Asian man was diagnosed with type 2 diabetes in 1984. He has required insulin treatment for the past five years and since diagnosis had developed diabetic nephropathy, diabetic neuropathy and preproliferative retinopathy. Past medical history included ischaemic heart disease, peripheral vascular disease, cerebrovascular disease and difficult-to-control hypertension (including hyperkalaemia with ACE inhibition). In 1986 he was diagnosed with abnormal haemoglobin consistent with variant AD. Fructosamine (reference range 200–285 µmol/l), rather than HbA_{1c}, was therefore checked as a marker of glycaemic control. Fructosamine predominantly represents glycation of albumin.

Treatment plan

IFCC 86mmol/mol ≡ DCCT 10.0%

In 2005, fructosamine was initially elevated at 440 µmol/l (measured IFCC HbA_{1c} 86 mmol/mol), with corresponding random laboratory glucose 15.8 mmol/l. In view of his progressive microvascular complications, the aim was to improve his glycaemic control and lower his fructosamine. Since 2005 the fructosamine values gradually decreased to 271 µmol/l in 2008

IFCC 74 ≡ DCCT 8.9%

(IFCC HbA_{1c} 74 mmol/mol), and random laboratory glucose 15.1 mmol/l. The clinical impression over this time was that glycaemic control had remained static despite the observed lower fructosamine results. This was based on home blood glucose (BM) monitoring, which showed acceptable fasting BM values (4.6–7.5 mmol/l) but progressive hyperglycaemia through the day (premeal BM 7–16 mmol/l). Over a similar timescale, urinary albumin:creatinine ratio (ACR) rose from 1.7 mg/mmol to 275 mg/mmol (normal range 0–3.5 mg/mmol). There were concerns that the fructosamine values did not reflect glycaemic control, so home blood glucose monitoring was used as the method of assessment.

Follow-up

Glycaemic control improved after input from the diabetes liaison team (BM 5–10 mmol/l). Last fructosamine was 273 µmol/l. Blood pressure was 140/72 mmHg and ACR had fallen to 93 mg/mmol following the addition of lisinopril 2.5 mg.

NICE Guidelines: Type 2 diabetes
HbA_{1c} targets: IFCC 48 mmol/mol ≡ 6.5% to IFCC 59 mmol/mol ≡ 7.5%

34: Recurrent hypoglycaemia caused by secondary adrenal insufficiency

Athinyaa Thiraviaraj, Hamza Ali Khan, Ailish G. Nugent and
G. Pooler R. Archbold, Specialist Registrars (AT, HAK), Consultant Physician (AGN), Consultant Chemical Pathologist (GPRA), Belfast, Northern Ireland, UK

Background

A 63-year-old man complained of recurrent hypoglycaemic episodes. He had been diagnosed 21 years previously with type 2 diabetes and had been insulin-requiring for 11 years. His diabetes was complicated by retinopathy, peripheral sensory neuropathy and Charcot's neuroarthropathy. For many years his IFCC HbA$_{1c}$ had been running about 97 mmol/mol, but by mid-2008 it had fallen to 64 and further to 51 mmol/mol by the end of 2008, despite a reduction in his dose of insulin from 86 units to 22 units daily. His diet had not changed and he had gained weight (BMI 37.1 kg/m²). His renal function was normal. There was a marked fall in blood pressure with posture (104/71 mmHg supine, and 80/57 mmHg standing).

IFCC 97 ≡ DCCT 11.0%
IFCC 64 ≡ DCCT 8.0%
IFCC 51 ≡ DCCT 6.8%

Adrenal insufficiency was suspected and was confirmed by a suboptimal short Synacthen test (baseline cortisol 156 nmol/l, 30-minute cortisol 392 nmol/l). ACTH was 18 ng/l. Further tests revealed free T$_4$ 7.1 pmol/l, TSH 2.257 mU/l, testosterone 2.2 nmol/l, FSH 2.9 U/l, LH 1.8 U/l, prolactin 575 mU/l (<400 mU/l), IGF-1 4.0 nmol/l (7–30 nmol/l). MRI of the pituitary gland showed a pituitary adenoma measuring 19×16 mm diameter. There was a moderate degree of suprasellar extension without impingement on to the optic chiasm.

Treatment and follow-up

The patient received hydrocortisone replacement and had no further episodes of hypoglycaemia. Postural hypotension improved but was still present, probably due to coexisting autonomic neuropathy. Thyroxine and testosterone replacement were started and the patient was referred for consideration for pituitary surgery.

NICE Guidelines: Type 2 diabetes
HbA$_{1c}$ targets: IFCC 48 mmol/mol ≡ 6.5% to IFCC 59 mmol/mol ≡ 7.5%

35: A patient with diabetes taking niacin

Richard Haynes and Jane Armitage, Clinical Research Fellow (RH),
Professor of Clinical Trials and Epidemiology (JA), Oxford, UK

Background

IFCC 50 ≡ DCCT 6.7%

A 63-year-old man was found to have type 2 diabetes at the time of a myocardial infarction in 2004. At the time of diagnosis his IFCC HbA_{1c} was 50 mmol/mol and he was managed with dietary advice. Despite treatment with atorvastatin 80 mg and ezetimibe 10 mg, his fasting lipid profile showed total cholesterol 4.7 mmol/l with LDL cholesterol 2.2 mmol/l, HDL cholesterol 0.8 mmol/l and triglycerides 3.7 mmol/l. He was intolerant of fenofibrate.

Treatment plan

IFCC 50 ≡ DCCT 6.7%
IFCC 62 ≡ DCCT 7.8%

In view of his persistently high LDL cholesterol and triglycerides, he was started on extended-release niacin at the local lipid clinic, which was titrated up to 2 g daily in line with product recommendations. He had some flushing with each dose increase, but this resolved. After two months on 2 g extended-release niacin, however, his IFCC HbA_{1c} had risen from 50 to 62 mmol/mol (a recognised complication of niacin therapy). His weight had remained stable and in view of the rise in his HbA_{1c} and history of coronary disease, metformin was added to his treatment, initially at 500 mg daily.

Follow-up

IFCC 62 ≡ DCCT 7.8%
IFCC 57 ≡ DCCT 7.4%
IFCC 55 ≡ DCCT 7.2%
IFCC 52 ≡ DCCT 6.9%
IFCC 54 ≡ DCCT 7.1%
IFCC 50 ≡ DCCT 6.7%
IFCC 60 ≡ DCCT 7.6%

The metformin dose was increased to 500 mg three times daily, and his IFCC HbA_{1c} fell from 62 to 57 mmol/mol. Subsequently over the next 18 months his IFCC HbA_{1c} was 55, 52 and 54 mmol/mol. His lipid profile improved to a total cholesterol of 3.9 mmol/l with LDL cholesterol 1.9 mmol/l, HDL cholesterol 1.0 mmol/l and triglycerides 2.2 mmol/l. He was regularly reviewed by his GP and his IFCC HbA_{1c} remained stable between 50 and 60 mmol/mol.

NICE Guidelines: Type 2 diabetes
HbA_{1c} targets: IFCC 48 mmol/mol ≡ 6.5% to IFCC 59 mmol/mol ≡ 7.5%

36: Tight glycaemic control leading to nocturnal hypoglycaemia

Rikke Borg, Research Fellow, Gentofte, Denmark

Background

A 47-year-old man had been diagnosed with type 1 diabetes at age 20. Since then he had attended the diabetes centre regularly, and showed no signs of diabetic retinopathy, nephropathy, or neuropathy. He was a non-smoker, had an active lifestyle, and his BMI was 24 kg/m². He was being treated with insulin aspart (29 units daily) by CSII (continuous subcutaneous insulin infusion) pump which he adjusted daily based on blood glucose monitoring. For years his HbA_{1c} levels had been low: IFCC HbA_{1c} 48–51 mmol/mol and eAG 7.7–8.2 mmol/l. Blood samples showed no signs of anaemia to cause low HbA_{1c}. He experienced mild hypoglycaemia several times a week, often in connection with physical exercise, and responded to these adequately with carbohydrate intake. He expressed a sense of well-being due to the tightly controlled low glucose levels.

IFCC 48 ≡ DCCT 6.5%
IFCC 51 ≡ DCCT 6.8%

As part of a local research project, he was offered continuous glucose monitoring (CGM) for periods of 48 hours. The CGM curve showed patterns of nocturnal periods of unrecognised hypoglycaemia, with glucose levels down to 2 mmol/l between 3 and 7 am.

Treatment plan

The first action was to lower the overnight basal insulin dose from 0.8 to 0.6 units/h. The following out-patient visits focused on education regarding the features of the pump, pausing the basal dose during exercise or hard work, and diminishing night-time doses if necessary. An occasional 3 am glucose measurement was introduced, and dietary consultations were arranged to discuss carbohydrate counting and how to anticipate physical activity. To avoid nocturnal hypoglycaemia, the future goal for IFCC HbA_{1c} was set at 53–59 mmol/mol, with eAG 8.5–9.3 mmol/l.

IFCC 53 ≡ DCCT 7.0%
IFCC 59 ≡ DCCT 7.5%

Follow-up

IFCC HbA_{1c} over the next year rose to 55, 56 and 54 mmol/mol (eAG: 8.9, 9.0, and 8.7 mmol/l). CGM identified the previously unrecognised hypoglycaemia and defined the vulnerable period overnight.

IFCC 55 ≡ DCCT 7.2%
IFCC 56 ≡ DCCT 7.3%
IFCC 54 ≡ DCCT 7.1%

NICE Guidelines: Type 1 diabetes in adults
HbA_{1c} targets: IFCC 48 mmol/mol ≡ 6.5% to IFCC 59 mmol/mol ≡ 7.5%

37: Diabetes and iron-deficiency anaemia

W. Garry John and Tara Wallace, Consultant Clinical Biochemist (WGJ),
Consultant Physician (TW), Norwich, UK

Background

A 42-year-old woman with a 20-year history of type 1 diabetes was seen in the diabetes clinic. She was on a basal bolus insulin regime consisting of insulin aspart (6 units before breakfast, 10 units before lunch and 14–20 units before evening meal) with insulin glargine (22 units before bed). She usually had good control with an IFCC HbA$_{1c}$ 53 mmol/mol, and on home blood glucose monitoring her capillary glucose levels were usually 4–6 mmol/l fasting, 4–7 mmol/l before lunch, 5–8 mmol/l before her evening meal and 7–11 mmol/l before bed. On this occasion, in clinic, her IFCC HbA$_{1c}$ had risen to 64 mmol/mol. There had been no change in her insulin dosage, no alterations to her diet or exercise regime and her home blood glucose readings were essentially unchanged. She reported only occasional episodes of mild hypoglycaemia with good hypoglycaemic awareness. She was well, apart from feeling a bit tired, and on questioning had suffered from menorrhagia for a year.

IFCC 53 ≡ DCCT 7.0%

IFCC 64 ≡ DCCT 8.0%

Treatment plan

Although HbA$_{1c}$ had risen, in view of her good home blood glucose readings, her insulin doses were not changed. Her haemoglobin level was found to be low at 9 g/dl; she also had low ferritin at 9 μg/l. She was started on ferrous sulphate replacement. Four months later a repeat ferritin determination was within the normal range at 32 μg/l. Her haemoglobin had risen to 12 g/dl and her IFCC HbA$_{1c}$ had fallen to 55 mmol/mol. Her home blood glucose levels were essentially unchanged.

IFCC 55 ≡ DCCT 7.2%

Follow up

It is important to recognise that iron deficiency anaemia has the affect of raising HbA$_{1c}$. The mechanism behind this increase is unknown, but may result in overtreatment if not recognised. It is interesting that the effect of iron-deficiency anaemia is more pronounced in patients with diabetes than in those without.

NICE Guidelines: Type 1 diabetes in adults
HbA$_{1c}$ targets: IFCC 48 mmol/mol ≡ 6.5% to IFCC 59 mmol/mol ≡ 7.5%

38: Deterioration in vision after commencing insulin treatment: the early worsening phenomenon

Peter H. Scanlon, Consultant Ophthalmologist, Cheltenham and Oxford, UK

Background

Type 2 diabetes was diagnosed in 1981 in an obese 41-year-old man, BMI 39 kg/m², and a diet recommended. His fasting glucose levels before HbA$_{1c}$ was measured, were 6–10 mmol/l. At the age of 48 years with his fasting glucose reaching 12 mmol/l, glibenclamide was introduced at 2.5 mg once daily and then increased gradually over the following 13 years to 15 mg. During this period, his fasting glucose levels were as before. Metformin was added at 500 mg twice daily, when the patient was aged 51 years. Aged 60 years, he developed circinate leakage of fatty deposits in his right eye and received focal laser treatment. His visual acuity (VA) was stable in both eyes at 6/9. One year later, aged 61 years, he developed an ulcer on his right foot. At this point his IFCC HbA$_{1c}$ was 89 mmol/mol.

IFCC 89 ≡ DCCT 10.3%

Treatment plan

His glibenclamide was stopped, insulin started and metformin continued. Within a few days of starting insulin, VA fell to 6/18 in the right eye and 6/24 in the left, and cystoid macular oedema (fluid accumulation within the macular area of the retina) was diagnosed. His IFCC HbA$_{1c}$ improved over the next three months, reaching 59 mmol/mol.

IFCC 59 = DCCT 7.5%

Follow-up

Over the next seven months, VA returned to 6/9 in each eye as the cystoid macular oedema resolved. Panretinal photocoagulation involving scatter laser to areas of the peripheral retina and vitrectomies, removal of vitreous humour, were performed 18 months later when the patient was aged 66 years to relieve the proliferative diabetic retinopathy. VA stabilised at 6/9 (right) and 6/60 (left) with left vision reduced due to ischaemic maculopathy (see Plate 2, page 75). His IFCC HbA$_{1c}$ remained below 64 mmol/mol.

IFCC 64 ≡ DCCT 8.0%

If a person has poor glycaemic control over the years, there is a risk of VA worsening initially on introduction of insulin. The long-term benefits of better glycaemic control, however, outweigh any short-term disadvantages. Good communication between the diabetologist and ophthalmologist is essential in this group of patients.

NICE Guidelines: Type 2 diabetes
HbA$_{1c}$ targets: IFCC 48 mmol/mol ≡ 6.5% to IFCC 59 mmol/mol ≡ 7.5%

39: Type 1 diabetes – worsening glycaemic control on introduction of a pump?

Ken Sikaris, Director of Chemical Pathology, Melbourne Pathology, Victoria, Australia

Background

A 13-year-old girl with type 1 diabetes for the past three years had moved from the childhood diabetes clinic to an adolescent clinic. Her diabetes had been well controlled using an insulin pen to inject short- or long-term insulin four times a day and her IFCC HbA_{1c} was 55 mmol/mol when last measured on a POCT device at the children's clinic.

IFCC 55 ≡ DCCT 7.2%

She had also started using an insulin pump for the last three months, where an interstitial needle (catheter) delivers short acting insulin at rates that can be adjusted to diet, activity, etc. Despite this advance in her treatment, her HbA_{1c} was tested in a private laboratory and the IFCC result of 64 mmol/mol was significantly worse, and above the target level of 58 mmol/mol.

IFCC 64 ≡ DCCT 8.0%
IFCC 58 ≡ DCCT 7.5%

Investigation

The family was concerned that her good diabetes control might have slipped now that she was on the insulin pump. The patient was also confused as she downloaded plasma glucose readings from both a continuous blood glucose monitoring device and a meter to proprietary software on the home PC, which indicated that her average glucose had not changed. Her average capillary plasma glucose readings while on the insulin pen were about 10 mmol/l (an IFCC HbA_{1c} 64 mmol/mol is equivalent to eAG of 10 mmol/l).

Follow-up

Two explanations are possible. There could be a difference in the way the POCT device and the private pathology laboratory measure HbA_{1c}. Calibration biases can occur and haemoglobin variants affect some methods of HbA_{1c} determination. This is most easily investigated by repeating the HbA_{1c} using an alternative method unaffected by haemoglobin variants.

The devices used for measuring glucose might not reflect average plasma glucose. This could be due to malfunction or because the daytime meter readings miss any nocturnal hypoglycaemia. This could be investigated by checking the devices with quality control samples and taking some readings on the meter overnight.

NICE Guidelines: Type 1 diabetes in children and young people
HbA_{1c} targets: IFCC <59 mmol/mol ≡ <7.5%

40: Monitoring glycaemic control in a patient with sickle cell trait

Andrea Gomes, Lis Chandler, Rachel Round and Janet Smith, on behalf of the GFH Study, Birmingham, UK

Background

A 23-year-old man of Yemeni origin attended a hospital diabetes clinic at University Hospital, Birmingham. He had been diagnosed with type 1 diabetes six years previously and had been treated with insulin. His BMI was 19.2 kg/m². There was no evidence of diabetic complications.

Investigation

The patient was a participant in a research study investigating the relationship between HbA_{1c}, fructosamine and glucose in patients with both variant haemoglobin and diabetes. Blood was obtained in the clinic by capillary sampling using a heparinised tube, and immediate measurement of glucose gave a random plasma glucose result of 20.0 mmol/l. Venous plasma glucose in a blood specimen taken later during a consultation for the research study and sent to the laboratory was 12.8 mmol/l. The accompanying serum fructosamine result was 413 μmol/l (reference range 200–285 μmol/l). Urinary ACR was <2.3 mg/mmol (<2.3 mg/mmol).

HPLC measurement of HbA_{1c} detected an additional peak in the S region. Another HPLC analyser used for identification of variant haemoglobin confirmed AS, sickle cell trait. The policy in this laboratory is not to report HbA_{1c} in patients with variant haemoglobin, however, for the purpose of the research study HbA_{1c} was determined by four different methods. IFCC HbA_{1c} was determined in heparinised capillary blood on Tosoh G8 HPLC analyser as 65 mmol/mol. EDTA blood samples were measured for IFCC HbA_{1c} with results of 72 from DCA 2000 analyser, 93 for Metrika A1cNOW+ cartridge (both immunochemical methods) and 67 mmol/mol for Primus Ultra2 affinity chromatography analyser. The patient had a normal haemoglobin level, (13.8 g/dl) and normal reticulocyte count (22.7×10^9/l (reference range 20–80/l).

IFCC 65 ≡ DCCT 8.1%
IFCC 72 ≡ DCCT 8.7%
IFCC 93 ≡ DCCT 10.7%
IFCC 67 ≡ DCCT 8.3%

Follow-up

Fructosamine is used rather than HbA_{1c} to monitor glycaemic control in this patient. HPLC measurement of HbA_{1c} should be used to detect variant haemoglobins in patients with diabetes, as their presence may affect HbA_{1c} results.

NICE Guidelines: Type 1 diabetes in children and young people
HbA_{1c} targets: IFCC 48 mmol/mol ≡ 6.5% to IFCC 59 mmol/mol ≡ 7.5%

41: Balancing fear of hypoglycaemia with optimal control in pregnancy

Roy Taylor, Professor of Medicine and Metabolism, Newcastle upon Tyne, UK

Background

A 19-year-old woman, diagnosed with type 1 diabetes at the age of 12, presented at 11 weeks' gestation with IFCC HbA$_{1c}$ 102 mmol/mol. Her HbA$_{1c}$ was satisfactory over the first few years after diagnosis on treatment with glargine and mealtime short-acting analogue insulin, (IFCC HbA$_{1c}$ 48-58 mmol/mol). Following a severe hypo at school, her glucose control had worsened (IFCC HbA$_{1c}$ 105 and 86 mmol/mol) and she had attended clinic infrequently.

IFCC 102 ≡ DCCT 11.5%
IFCC 48 ≡ DCCT 6.5%
IFCC 58 ≡ DCCT 7.5%
IFCC 105 ≡ DCCT 11.8%
IFCC 86 ≡ DCCT 10.0%

Treatment plan

With little change in prescribed insulin dose, her HbA$_{1c}$ fell (IFCC HbA$_{1c}$ 81, 56 and 53 mmol/mol at 16, 20 and 24 weeks) and she treated occasional mild hypos herself without difficulty. A severe hypo at 26 weeks led to her decreasing doses of glargine to reduce the risk of hypos. She remained very fearful of recurring hypos and her HbA$_{1c}$ rose (IFCC HbA$_{1c}$ 62 mmol/mol at 28 weeks). Her fasting blood glucose (FBG) target range was revised to 4.5–7.0 mmol/l to balance the risk of hypo against the effects of high blood glucose on the baby, but her control remained poor (FBG >7 mmol/l and IFCC HbA$_{1c}$ 59 and 64 mmol/mol) until delivery by Caesarian section of a 4.3 kg baby at 38 weeks.

IFCC 81 ≡ DCCT 9.6%
IFCC 56 ≡ DCCT 7.3%
IFCC 53 ≡ DCCT 7.0%
IFCC 62 ≡ DCCT 7.8%

IFCC 59 ≡ DCCT 7.5%
IFCC 64 ≡ DCCT 8.0%

Follow-up

IFCC HbA$_{1c}$ was 78 mmol/mol at her postnatal visit six weeks after delivery. Contact was lost until nine weeks into her second pregnancy (IFCC HbA$_{1c}$ 86 mmol/mol), which was terminated due to multiple fetal abnormalities. After a further 18 months, under more stable domestic circumstances, she re-presented, determined to improve the control of her diabetes before attempting conception again. IFCC HbA$_{1c}$ improved from 63 to 48–53 mmol/mol. High dose folic acid was started. IFCC HbA$_{1c}$ was 45 mmol/mol at conception and averaged 48 and 52 mmol/mol during the second and third trimesters. A normal 3.7 kg baby was born at 38 weeks. The mother's IFCC HbA$_{1c}$ six weeks after delivery was 58 mmol/mol. A stable home life is a powerful determinant of HbA$_{1c}$.

IFCC 78 ≡ DCCT 9.3%

IFCC 86 ≡ DCCT 10.0%

IFCC 63 ≡ DCCT 7.9%
IFCC 48 ≡ DCCT 6.5%
IFCC 53 ≡ DCCT 7.0%
IFCC 45 ≡ DCCT 6.3%
IFCC 52 ≡ DCCT 6.9%
IFCC 58 ≡ DCCT 7.5%

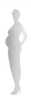

NICE Guidelines: Diabetes in pregnancy
HbA$_{1c}$ target prepregnancy*: IFCC <43 mmol/mol ≡ <6.1%
*(if safely achievable)

42: Asian patient with high-risk feet and suboptimal glycaemic control

Varadarajan Baskar, Consultant Physician, Wolverhampton, UK

Background

A 74-year-old man of Indo-Asian descent was referred to the high-risk foot clinic with peripheral neuropathy and progressive intermittent claudication. He was known to have had type 2 diabetes since 2003; treated with metformin 1 g twice daily. He had no known cardiovascular complications; he had stopped smoking several years before and did not consume any alcohol. His BMI was 24 kg/m² and his blood pressure 142/79 mmHg. Foot examination confirmed peripheral neuropathy and absent left foot pulses, and there were no audible vascular bruits. Blood profile at review was IFCC HbA$_{1c}$ 93 mmol/mol, serum creatinine 88 μmol/l, eGFR 77 ml/min, total cholesterol 5.2 mmol/l, HDL cholesterol 1.4 mmol/l and TSH 1.30 mU/l. His normal haemoglobin (13.9 g/dl) and MCV (94 fl) excluded significant haemoglobinopathy.

IFCC 93 ≡ DCCT 10.7%

Treatment plan

In view of established peripheral vascular disease with progressive and significant claudication, it was felt that he would benefit from a full vascular assessment and review. Follow-up from the high-risk foot clinic plus education on self-care was recommended. His poorly-controlled diabetes on metformin monotherapy needed additional treatment to attain the target IFCC HbA$_{1c}$ of 53 mmol/mol; whereas his lipid profile with established peripheral vascular disease and diabetes needed treatment with simvastatin 40 mg once daily. Borderline elevated blood pressure should be re-checked with a view to intervention if systolic result persistently remained >140 mmHg.

IFCC 53 ≡ DCCT 7.0%

Follow-up

He had angioplasty to his left femoral artery with good improvement in his claudication distance. Gliclazide was started at 80 mg once daily and progressively titrated up to a dose of 160 mg twice daily over the subsequent six months. His IFCC HbA$_{1c}$ at 3, 6 and 12 months after review had improved to 76, 69 and 61 mmol/mol. His lipid profile improved (total cholesterol 4.1 mmol/l) and systolic blood pressure stayed at <140 mmHg on subsequent re-checks without treatment.

IFCC 76 ≡ DCCT 9.1%
IFCC 69 ≡ DCCT 8.5%
IFCC 61 ≡ DCCT 7.7%

NICE Guidelines: Type 2 diabetes
HbA$_{1c}$ targets: IFCC 48 mmol/mol ≡ 6.5% to IFCC 59 mmol/mol ≡ 7.5%

43: Type 2 diabetes and polycystic ovarian syndrome

M. Ali Karamat, Clinical Lecturer in Diabetes and Endocrinology,
Birmingham, UK

Background

A 29-year-old woman was diagnosed with type 2 diabetes in 2003. She had no osmotic symptoms of diabetes but had a high BMI at 39 kg/m². She developed gestational diabetes during pregnancy in 2001 and was on insulin four times daily. A 3.4 kg girl was delivered by emergency Caesarean section at around 38 weeks. She was also noted to have autoimmune hypothyroidism and polycystic ovarian syndrome as other relevant conditions. She was on replacement doses of 75 µg thyroxine and thyroid function tests were normal, with FT4 of 15.3 pmol/l and TSH of 2.56 mIU/l. Her blood pressure was reasonably well controlled at 131/86 mmHg and urinary ACR was normal at 0.2 mg/mmol.

Treatment plan

IFCC 53 ≡ DCCT 7.0%

IFCC 48 ≡ DCCT 6.5%

She was seen in the pre-conception clinic as she and her partner wanted to try for a further pregnancy. In view of her BMI, appropriate first-line treatment would be metformin with advice on diet and lifestyle. It was noted at clinic review that her BMI was 41 kg/m². IFCC HbA$_{1c}$ was 53 mmol/mol. In view of her intended pregnancy, she was recommended to aim for a more tight control, toward IFCC HbA$_{1c}$ of 48 mmol/mol. Because of potential teratogenic potential of drugs like ACE inhibitors and statins she was not started on these drugs.

Follow-up

IFCC 53 ≡ DCCT 7.0%

The patient was counselled with lifestyle and dietary advice and started on metformin 500 mg once daily, which was then titrated to 500 mg twice daily to aim for tighter control. Her IFCC HbA$_{1c}$ was still 53 mmol/mol. Regular follow-up was advised as it was extremely likely that she would require insulin during pregnancy, with the hormonal changes that occur particularly during the second half of pregnancy.

NICE Guidelines: Type 2 diabetes
HbA$_{1c}$ targets: IFCC 48 mmol/mol ≡ 6.5% to IFCC 59 mmol/mol ≡ 7.5%

44: Impact of variant haemoglobin AC on HbA$_{1c}$ determination

Laura Hikin, Jackie Carr-Smith, Rachel Round and Janet Smith, on behalf of the GFH Study, University Hospital Birmingham, Birmingham, UK

Background

An Asian woman aged 74 years attended a diabetes outpatient clinic in the West Midlands. She had been diagnosed with type 2 diabetes 21 years previously and was treated with insulin and oral hypoglycaemic agents. Her BMI was 33.4 kg/m^2. She was hypertensive and had never smoked. She had retinopathy but no evidence of nephropathy, neuropathy or macrovascular complications.

Investigation

The patient consented to join a research study to investigate the relationships between different markers of glycaemic control i.e. HbA$_{1c}$, fructosamine and random plasma glucose in patients with both variant haemoglobin and diabetes. A variant haemoglobin, AC, had previously been identified by the haematology department. She had a normal reticulocyte count, 44 x10^9/l (reference range 20–80), slightly low Hb at 10.7 g/dl (11.5–16.5) and microcytosis, with mean cell volume of 68.6 fl (78–98 fl) and mean cell haemoglobin 22.9 pg (27.0–33.0 pg). The random plasma glucose obtained initially in the clinic by immediate measurement of a capillary sample was 12.1 mmol/l. Later at a consultation for the research study, it was 11.0 mmol/l on a venous fluoride oxalate sample sent to the laboratory for analysis.

An additional peak was detected using HPLC (Tosoh G8 analyser) confirming HbAC heterozygosity and IFCC HbA$_{1c}$ determined as 96 mmol/mol. This result would not have been reported routinely for a patient with variant haemoglobin, in line with the policy of the laboratory. When HbA$_{1c}$ was measured by other techniques, the IFCC results recorded were 97 for DCA 2000 analyser, >118 for Metrika A$_{1c}$NOW+ cartridge (both immunochemical methods) and 89 mmol/mol for Primus Ultra2 affinity chromatography analyser.

IFCC 96 ≡ DCCT 10.9%

IFCC 97 ≡ DCCT 11.0%
IFCC 118 ≡ DCCT 12.9%
IFCC 89 ≡ DCCT 10.3%

Follow-up

HbA$_{1c}$ was not used to monitor glycaemic control in this patient due to the presence of variant haemoglobin. Instead fructosamine, which reflects glycaemic control over the previous two weeks, was used to monitor glycaemic control as she had normal albumin excretion.

NICE Guidelines: Type 2 diabetes
HbA$_{1c}$ targets: IFCC 48 mmol/mol ≡ 6.5% to IFCC 59 mmol/mol ≡ 7.5%

45: Diabetic nephropathy

Sally M. Marshall, Professor of Diabetes, Newcastle upon Tyne, UK

Background

A woman had developed type 1 diabetes in 1954, aged 10 years. In 1985 she required laser treatment for proliferative retinopathy. She had a myocardial infarction in 1992, with coronary artery bypass grafting in 1998. Proteinuria was first noted in 1991 and despite good blood pressure control with lisinopril, serum creatinine rose progressively from 90 µmol/l (eGFR 58 ml/min/1.73 m^2) in 1991 to 230 µmol/l (eGFR 18 ml/min/1.73 m^2) in 2009. Glycaemic control was suboptimal, with IFCC HbA$_{1c}$ running between 75–86 mmol/mol, on twice-daily pre-mixed insulin. However, the woman was adamant that she did not wish to intensify glycaemic control.

IFCC 75 ≡ DCCT 9.0%
IFCC 86 ≡ DCCT 10.0%

Treatment plan

In 2007 she complained of tiredness. Haemoglobin was 9.4 g/dl, MCV 72 fl and ferritin 16 µg/l. After iron supplementation, erythropoietin therapy was started. After six months, haemoglobin was 11.2 g/dl and eGFR remained stable (24 ml/min/1.73 m^2). Insulin therapy and self-monitored blood glucose (SMBG) levels were unchanged and there was no increased hypoglycaemia. However, IFCC HbA$_{1c}$ fell from 83 to 58 mmol/mol.

IFCC 83 ≡ DCCT 9.7%
IFCC 58 ≡ DCCT 7.5%

Red blood cell turnover is abnormal in chronic kidney disease. The high HbA$_{1c}$ reflects longer red cell survival, with increased glycation. With erythropoietin, there is an increase in the number of young red cells and HbA$_{1c}$ falls.

Follow-up

In 2009, the woman began to experience frequent episodes of hypoglycaemia, some severe and requiring third party help. SMBG levels were frequently <4.0 mmol/l. IFCC HbA$_{1c}$ had fallen further, to 48 mmol/mol and eGFR to 18 ml/min/1.73 m^2. The dose of twice daily pre-mixed insulin was reduced in steps from 36+22 units to 18+12 units per 24h. The woman remained adamant that she would not consider an alternative insulin regimen. She was advised that the reduction in dose was necessary because the failing kidneys were unable to excrete insulin not metabolised in her body.

IFCC 48 ≡ DCCT 6.5%

NICE Guidelines: Type 1 diabetes in adults
HbA$_{1c}$ targets: IFCC 48 mmol/mol ≡ 6.5% to IFCC 59 mmol/mol ≡ 7.5%

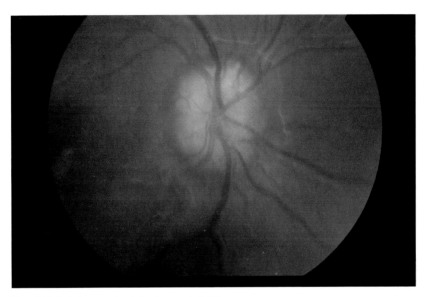

Plate 1 Retinal photograph relating to case study 29.

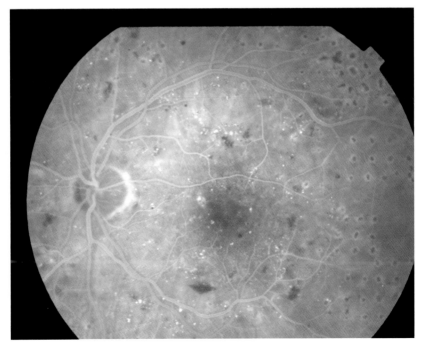

Plate 2 Retinal photograph relating to case study 38. Note the enlarged foveal avascular zone with an irregular contour, consistent with ischaemic maculopathy.

Conversion table for HbA$_{1c}$ from IFCC to DCCT-aligned units

IFCC HbA$_{1c}$ (mmol/mol)	DCCT HbA$_{1c}$ (%)
20	4.0
25	4.4
30	4.9
35	5.4
40	5.8
45	6.3
50	6.7
55	7.2
60	7.6
65	8.1
70	8.6
75	9.0
80	9.5
85	9.9
90	10.4
95	10.8
100	11.3
110	12.2
120	13.1
130	14.0
140	15.0
150	15.9

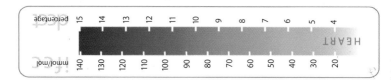

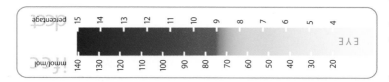

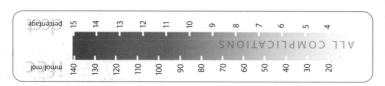

Thermometers relating HbA$_{1c}$ to the complications of type 2 diabetes.